Waldemar Ch. Hecker

Surgical Correction of Intersexual Genitalia and Female Genital Malformation

With a Section on Pediatric Endocrinology
by Dieter Knorr

Translation by Terry C. Telger

With 27 Figures
in 82 Separate Illustrations

Springer-Verlag
Berlin Heidelberg NewYork Tokyo

Prof. Dr. WALDEMAR CH. HECKER

Prof. Dr. DIETER KNORR

Kinderchirurgische Klinik im
Dr. von Haunerschen Kinderspital
der Universität München
Lindwurmstraße 4
8000 München 2

Translator:

Mr. TERRY C. TELGER
6112 Waco Way, Fort Worth
TX 76133/USA

ISBN-13:978-3-642-70366-9 e-ISBN-13:978-3-642-70364-5
DOI: 10.1007/978-3-642-70364-5

Library of Congress Cataloging in Publication Data. Hecker, W. Christian (Waldemar Christian). Surgical correction of intersexual genitalia and female genital malformation. Translation of: Operative Korrekturen des intersexuellen und des fehlgebildeten weiblichen Genitales. Bibliography: p. Includes index.
1. Generative organs – Abnormalities – Surgery. 2. Generative organs, Female – Abnormalities – Surgery. 3. Sex differentiation disorders – Surgery. 4. Sex differentiation disorders – Endocrine aspects. 5. Pediatric endocrinology. 6. Children – Surgery. I. Knorr, Dieter. II. Title. [DNLM: 1. Endocrine Diseases – diagnosis. 2. Genitalia, Female – abnormalities. 3. Genitalia, Female – surgery. 4. Sex Differentiation Disorders – diagnosis. 5. Sex Differentiation Disorders – surgery. WJ 712 H4490] RD584.H4313 1985 618.1′45 85-8143

Reproduction of the figures: Gustav Dreher GmbH, Stuttgart

2123/3130-543210

Preface

This book is the product of long years of close collaboration between two physicians, a pediatric endocrinologist and a pediatric surgeon, who are interested in the complex field of human malformations. Their efforts have set a new standard in the treatment of children with intersexual or malformed female genitalia.

It is impossible to convey the details of complex surgical procedures without the help of meticulous illustrations. It is fortunate that happened to meet an academically trained artist, Mrs. Siri Mills, M.A., while visiting in the United States. Her excellent knowledge of anatomy, her remarkable skills as an artist and technical illustrator, and her readiness to include all details of interest to the surgeon have found their fruitful expression in the illustrations of this book.

We express our thanks to Springer-Verlag and especially to Prof. Dietrich Goetze, at whose suggestion this book was written, for their amiable compliance with all our wishes, and particularly for their willingness to retain Mrs. Mills as our illustrator.

Munich, May 1985 WALDEMAR HECKER

Contents

Part 2: Surgical Measures for the Correction of Intersexual Genitalia and Female Genital Malformations

AGS	congenital adrenogenital syndrome
CAH	congenital adrenal hyperplasia
HCG	human chorionic gonadotropin
HMG	Human menopausal gonadotropin
RIA	Radioimmunoassay

Introduction

Intersexuality has fascinated mankind since antiquity and has been a popular subject in art, as evidenced by hundreds of statues and drawings from early Greek culture.

One of the "deans" of German pediatric surgeons, Dr. Fritz Rehbein of Bremen, recounts the following legend based upon his studies of androgyny:

Hermaphroditos, the bisexual godling, was the son of Hermes and Aphrodite. Reared by the nyphms of Mount Ida near Troy, the boy left his mountain home at the age of 15 and journeyed through Asia Minor. There he came to Caria and the spring of the fountain-nymph Salmacis, who was combing her long hair as she watched her reflection in the water. When she saw the youth she fell madly in love with him, but he rejected her advances. Later, when Salmacis saw the boy bathing in her spring, she forcibly embraced him, and the gods answered her prayer by fusing their bodies into one. Hermaphroditos was now a true hermaphrodite, a female boy.

Rehbein speculates that Hermaphroditos is probably the mythological expression of a deity which is sexually undifferentiated, and which also may be viewed as a relic from the early stage of maternal religion, which ascribes male attributes to the great goddess or assigns to her a masculine counterpart in the form of a hero.

Rehbein further suggests that androgynous deities were a very early prototype of the personal concept of God and survived as such in myths. Only in later, more advanced cultures did the masculine concept of the deity become established. Rehbein concludes his studies with the reminder that all of us are intersexual in the earliest stage of embryonic development, and that every human being carries remnants of the other sex throughout his lifetime. Expressed in mythologic terms, one might say that for a few weeks we all experience a precosmic state in which "opposites" are in balance, analogous to the fusion of the "world parents" in a Japanese creation myth, and must recapitulate the genesis of a cosmos or microcosmos. Certainly the ancients were impressed and inspired by the sight of a human being in whom sexual differentiation was absent or anomalous. Perhaps they regarded this being as the manifestation of a creative deity in its original form.

We do not know whether these ancient hermaphrodites were happy. We do know that hermaphroditism causes profound unhappiness today, and that the condition is an indication for psychological referral. We believe that the healthy emotional development of the intersexual individual depends upon a normalization of his external appearance, and thus upon the surgical correction of his ambiguous genitals combined with appropriate endocrine therapy.

Part 1
Endocrinologic Diagnosis in Pediatric Patients with Genital Anomalies

General Rules

The purpose of this chapter is to aid the pediatric surgeon in his decision-making. It is not a substitute for endocrinologic or genetic consultation in specific cases.

The diagnosis of genital anomalies must be approached with the utmost care, for the results will decide, often irrevocably, whether the patient will be happy or unhappy in his future sexual life. Corrective surgery of the genitals and definitive sex assignment should be done as early in life as possible so that the child will not have to cope consciously with his genital abnormality or sexually ambiguous status. While it was once believed that surgical intervention should be delayed until puberty to see how the child would develop somatically and psychosexually, this practice is no longer considered appropriate, for even small children must have an opportunity to identify with their somatic sex. A sex reversal after the age of 3 years will have profound psychologic and social effects on the patient and the family.

Before corrective surgery is performed, it is necessary to complete all endocrinologic and genetic studies, even if they are more time-consuming than the operation itself. While impatience on the part of the parents and surgeon is understandable, hasty surgical measures may cause irreversible harm. Because errors are always possible, we require two independent test results for all critical investigations, such as karyography in mixed gonadal dysgenesis, which will dictate the need for bilateral gonadectomy.

With modern endocrinologic investigations and stimulation tests, it is possible to predict with a high degree of confidence the hormonal development of intersexual children during puberty, and thus to guide the pediatric surgeon is selecting the "right" operation for a given patient. Occasionally situations will arise in which the sex that is selected for a child differs from its gonadal or chromosomal sex. In making such a decision, it is imperative that the parents be thoroughly advised as to the sexual and medical implications of the procedure. In addition, they must stand behind their decision without reservation to ensure that the child will acquire its intended sexual identity and not be exposed to conflicting signals.

Not all genital anomalies can be surgically corrected with a perfect cosmetic result. Many parents attempt to hide the fact of a genital abnormality from their child for as long as possible, believing that the child will be better able to deal with the knowledge at an older age. Such behavior is understandable but misguided. Children are quick to sense "strangeness" of their genitals even at a very early age. The child who has approached his parents with a question about his genital problems and been rebuffed is not likely to raise the subject again and will bear his anxiety alone. The responsibility of informing the child at an early age is especially keen in cases of confirmed infertility. The young child will assimilate this information slowly and calmly and will grow without difficulty into his inescapable role. Waiting until puberty or later adolescence to disclose a long-known infertility to the young patient will inevitably cause psychological trauma and precipitate a crisis of trust toward parents and physicians.

I will never forget a 14-year-old girl with Ullrich-Turner syndrome who, when finally told of her condition, screamed at her parents. "I've known for a long time, but why didn't you tell me before? How could you be so mean?"

Endocrinology of Antenatal Sex Differentiation

Male Differentiation

In the first weeks after fertilization, the primitive gonads differ in their karyotype as 46 XX or 46 XY, but they do not yet differ histologically. By week 7 of embryonic life the primitive male gonad begins to differentiate along masculine lines under the influence of a factor called "HY antigen."

By week 8 the embryonic testis begins to secrete testosterone. At this time both the müllerian ducts and the wolffian urinary ducts are still present.

Under the influence of embryonic testosterone production the wolffian duct system differentiates further into the epididymis, ductus deferens, seminal vesicles, and anterior part of the prostate. The testosterone exerts its effect on the target organs only if it is specifically bound by a receptor globulin in the cells of those organs. As development progresses, the embryonic and fetal testis elaborates a glycoprotein which causes the müllerian duct system to atrophy. This glycoprotein is called the "müllerian duct inhibiting factor" or "oviduct repressor."

During week 12 the embryonic urethral groove closes under the influence of embryonic testosterone to form the male urethra. Regular closure of the urethral groove and a normal fetal development of the male penis require that the endogenous testosterone be metabolized to 5α-dihydrotestosterone by an enzyme of 5α-reductase in these target organs.

Female Differentiation

While male sex differentiation relies on a series of active hormonal processes, female sex differentiation is passive and occurs in the absence of masculinizing hormonal events, regardless of the chromosomal sex. Only the later differentiation of the ovaries requires the existence of at least two X chromosomes.

If the wolffian ducts are not stimulated by testosterone they gradually regress. If the müllerian ducts are not repressed by the testicular inhibiting factor they continue to develop, forming the uterus and tubes. Opinions differ as to whether the cranial vagina also arises from the müllerian ducts. As Jost has shown, the internal and external genitalia will differentiate along feminine lines even if the gonads are absent.

The role played by hormonal psychosexual "imprinting" in human beings is uncertain. Such a phenomenon has definitely been shown to exist in rodents.

Specific Endocrinologic Diagnosis and Therapy

Virilization of the Female External Genitalia

Documentation. The degree of virilization of the female external genitalia is classified internationally according to the scheme of Prader (Fig. 1).

Congenital Adrenogenital Syndrome with a Defect of 21-Hydroxylase

The congenital adrenogenital snydrome (AGS), called also congenital adrenal hyperplasia (CAH), is the most frequent cause of virilization of the female external genitalia. It is transmitted as an autosomal recessive trait and has a prevalence of about 1:7000 to 12000.

Definitive Test. Radioimmunoassay of plasma 17α-hydroxyprogesterone is diagnostic.

Normal values after the neonatal period:	50–300 ng/dl
17OH-Progesterone in AGS:	3000–70000 ng/dl

During the neonatal period, and especially in premature infants, nonspecific elevations of 17OH-progesterone are found. The results of the 17OH-

Fig. 1. Prader's classification of the morphology of the external genitalia. Left column: *Normal male and female types;* right column: *intermediate stages ranging (top to bottom) from the near-normal female (type 1) to the near-normal male (type 5)*

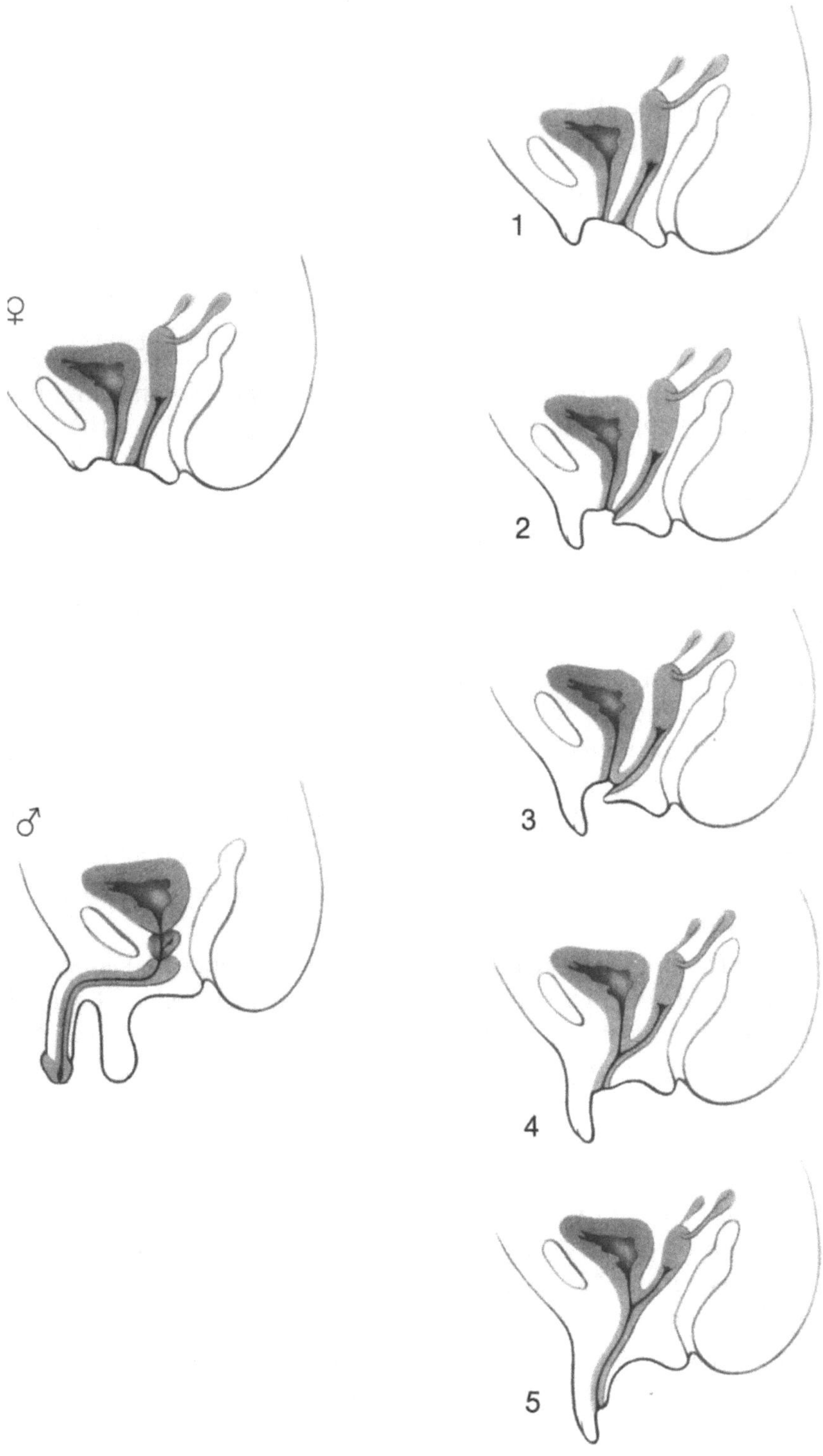
♀
♂
1
2
3
4
5

progesterone assay should always be confirmed by repeating the assay after the 5th week of life.

Specific results are also provided by the assay of urinary pregnanetriol and pregnanetriolone after the neonatal period.

Normal values:

Pregnanetriolone:	Not demonstrated	
Pregnanetriol:	Infant:	up to 300 μg/day
	Preschool child:	50–500 μg/day
	School-age child:	100–1000 μg/day
	Adult:	400–4000 μg/day

With an untreated 21-hydroxylase defect, pregnanetriolone can always be demonstrated. Pregnanetriol excretion is increased to 5000–100000 μg/day.

Assay of steroid metabolites in the urine is also useful for the diagnosis of other, far less common forms of AGS, such as an 11-hydroxylase defect or 3β-hydroxysteroid dehydrogenase defect. The classic 21-hydroxylase defect is so characteristic biochemically that assays obviate the need for karyography in patients with intersexual genitals.

The 21-hydroxylase deficit may assume any of three clinical forms, which represent genetic entities; this means that a particular form is almost always seen in a particular family.

The most severe from is congenital salt-losing syndrome. At one time, affected children invariably died in infancy from hyponatremia and hyperkalemia. Patients with this syndrome require glucocorticoid and mineralocorticoid replacement for life. Girls with the syndrome have intersexual external genitals at birth, usually of Prader type III–V.

A milder form of the 21-hydroxylase defect is uncomplicated adrenogenital syndrome. Affected girls may have Prader type I–III external genitalia. In other cases the syndrome is not recognized until early childhood, when clitoral hypertrophy and premature pubic hair growth are noted.

The third, mildest form of the 21-hydroxylase defect has been recognized as a genetic entity only in recent years and is referred to as the "cryptic" or "late-onset" form. This defect may be revealed by incidental biochemical testing during familial examinations (cryptic), or it may be manifested by virilization during puberty (late onset).

In all girls with AGS, the internal genitals are strictly female, i.e., the uterine adnexa and ovaries are always present.

As a rule, girls with AGS should be reared in their gonadal sex. A possible exception is Prader type V antenatal virilization with the development of a large, penis-like clitoris. Because the nonkeratinizing squamous epithelium of the vulva is absent in such patients and a good "male member" is present, it may be preferable to rear the child as a male, especially if the child has already been reared in that sex for several years. Of course, an oophorectomy must also be elected in such cases. Because this syndrome is always of the salt-losing variety fertility is seldom achieved, even in children who are reared as females.

Pharmacologic Therapy. All forms of congenital AGS are based upon a defect of cortisol biosynthesis. Thus, differentiated glucocorticoid and possibly mineralocorticoid replacement take priority over corrective surgery. This therapy must be maintained for life to prevent further virilization. Under the stress of surgery it is important that the dosage be temporarily increased. Discontinuing corticoid therapy to "fast" the patient for surgery would constitute serious negligence!

Other causes of antenatal virilization in girls are rare compared with AGS. These include maternal ingestion of androgenic drugs during pregnancy (anabolic 19-nortestosterone) and the presence of maternal androgen-secreting adrenal or ovarian tumors. Maternal virilization in such cases may be relatively mild.

Postnatal virilization in girls may be associated with massive clitoral hypertrophy but cannot produce a urogenital sinus malformation.

Intersexual Genitals Due to Deficient Androgenization of the Male

Defects of Testosterone Biosynthesis

Even forms of penile hypospadias (grade 2) are often characterized by an insufficient rise of plasma testosterone in the HCG test, indicating subnormal testosterone levels during embryonic life as a possible cause of the anomaly (Figs. 2 and 3).

In scrotal and perineal hypospadias, 36% of patients show a subnormal testosterone response to HCG.

All forms of impaired testosterone biosynthesis based on an autosomal recessive enzyme defect (38-hydroxysteroid dehydrogenase defect, 17-hydroxylase defect, 17/20-desmolase defect, 17-hydroxysteroid dehydrogenase defect, 5α-reductase defect) present the clinical picture of male pseudohermaphroditism, i.e., a normal male karyotype with ambiguous or purely female genitalia.

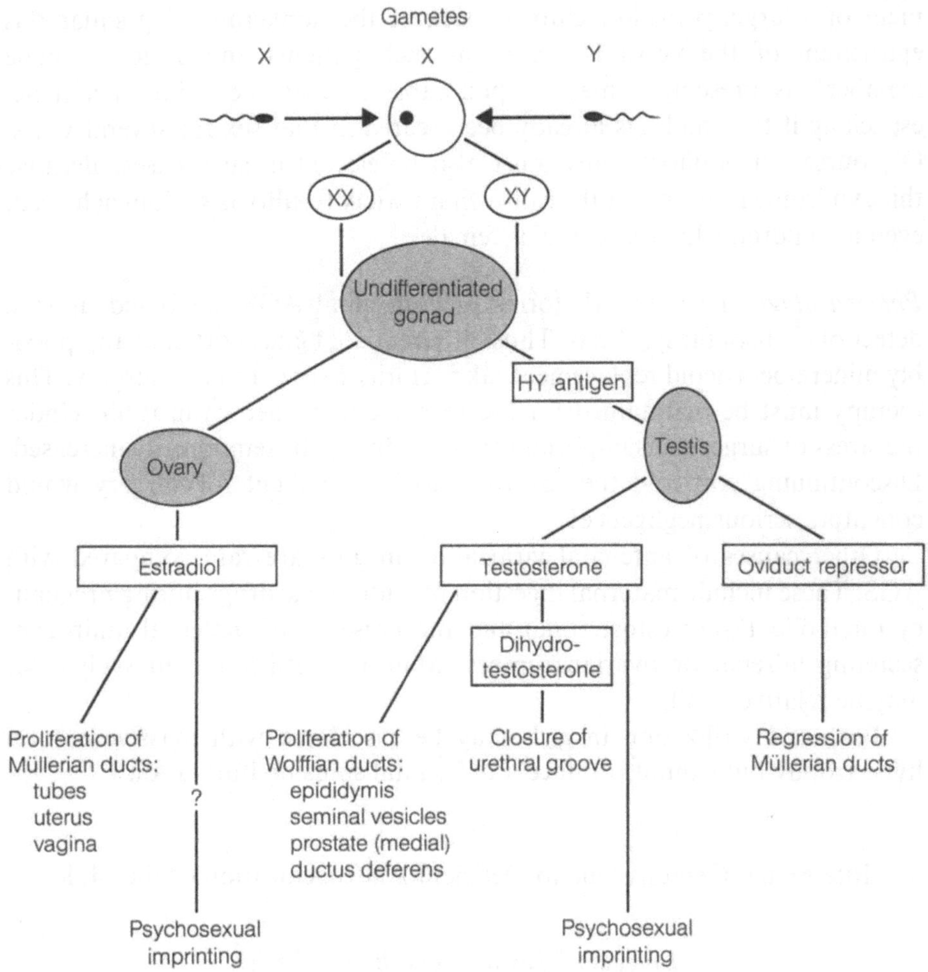

Fig. 2. The endocrinologic features of antenatal sex differentiation

When assigning the sex of rearing, one must be guided by the patient's gonadal function, anatomy, and prognosis. While enzyme defects up to the testosterone stage will not improve with time, boys with a 5α-reductase defect may be expected to undergo full virilization at puberty.

Another peculiarity is the pronounced pubertal breast development that occurs in patients with a 17-hydroxysteroid oxydoreductase defect. Almost all patients with this defect are reared as females.

In all forms of impaired androgenization except type 1 or 2 hypospadias with conspicuous testes, the karyogram must be obtained before surgery is performed.

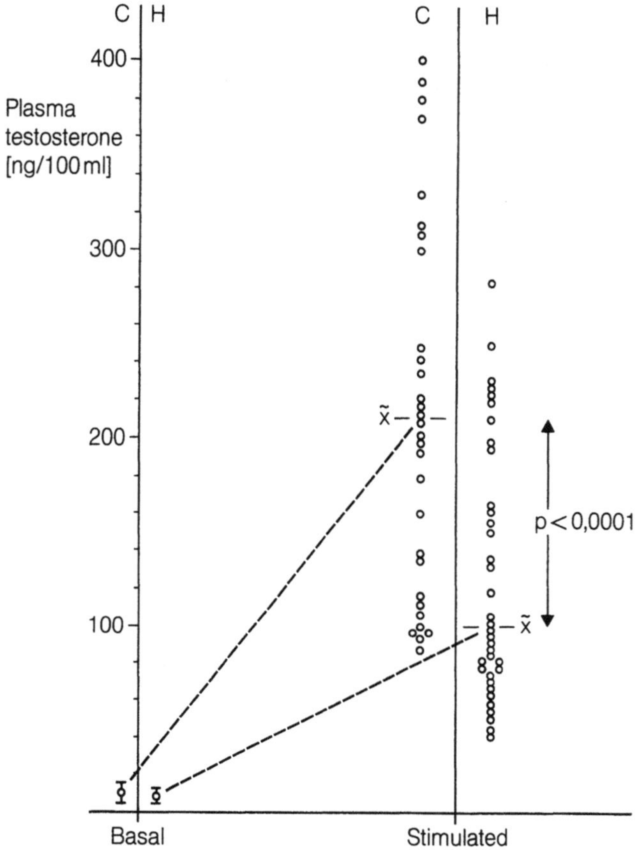

Fig. 3. Rise of plasma testosterone over a 3-day period following a single administration of 5000 units HCG in "controls" (boys with undescended testes) (C) *and in boys with grade 2–4 hypospadias* (H)

Androgen Receptor Defects

A special form of deficient masculinization in the male is testicular feminization.

In complete testicular feminization the external genitalia appear to be female. However, the vagina is rudimentary and ends in a blind pouch 1–2 cm deep. The uterus is absent. Frequently the patient presents with unilateral or bilateral inguinal hernias, which at surgery are found to contain testes. Axillary and pubic hair is extremely sparse ("hairless women"), and primary amenorrhea is present. Incomplete forms with intersexual genitals also occur.

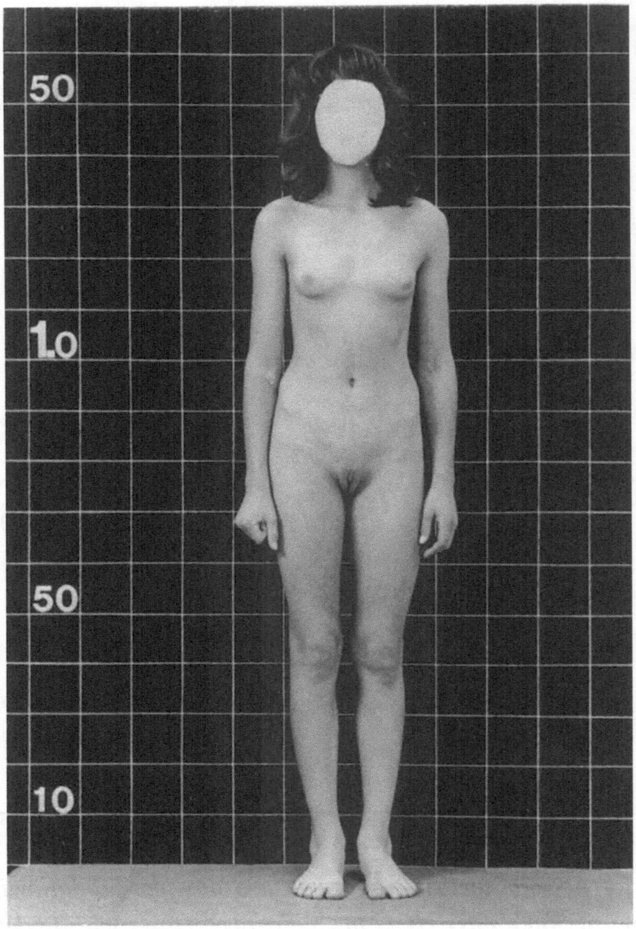

Fig. 4. "Girl" 15 years of age with untreated testicular feminization (46 XY karyotype). The patient was operated on for inguinal hernias in infancy. Plasma testosterone is 1200 ng/dl. An "aunt" has the same disorder

Diagnosis. The diagnosis is established by:

The presence of other apparent females with primary amenorrhea in the maternal line

Male plasma testosterone levels (50–300 ng/dl) in the 2nd and 3rd months of life without stimulation

The demonstration of extremely high testosterone levels in the presence of primary amenorrhea past the age of puberty

A demonstrated failure of testosterone binding to cells of testosterone-dependent organs (e.g., the genital skin)

These young "women" have two to three times higher testosterone levels than adult men (1000–2000 ng/dl) but show no evidence of virilization (Fig. 4).

A presumptive diagnosis of testicular feminization can usually be made from the clinical picture of an XY female with testis-containing inguinal hernias and a blind vaginal pouch. The HCG test elicits a male-type stimulation of testosterone values, even before the age of puberty. The breasts of these patients are well developed despite the absence of ovaries.

Cause. The target organs fail to respond to testosterone because they lack the specific testosterone receptor globulin. The defect is probably inherited as an X-linked recessive trait. Although a male 46 XY karyotype is present and testes may be demonstrated, it is imperative that these patients be allowed to retain their female identity. However, a prophylactic gonadectomy is recommended after the age of puberty, in view of the 30% incidence of gonadoblastoma in females under 30. A total vaginoplasty in patients who lack a rudimentary vagina should not be considered until the patient wishes to become sexually active; otherwise the danger of stenosis is too great.

Gonadectomy must be followed by chronic estrogen replacement, e.g., oral ethinylestradiol at a dose of 0.02 mg/day.

Persistence of the Müllerian Ducts

The müllerian ducts regress completely in the male during embryonic life under the influence of müllerian duct inhibiting factor (oviduct repressor), a protein elaborated by the testis.

When there is a defect of this inhibiting factor, the müllerian duct system continues to develop along feminine lines, forming tubes and a uterus. Because testosterone is also being produced if testes are present, the wolffian ducts also differentiate into sperm-conveying structures. These structures are invariably abnormal as a result of anatomic competition. Abdominal cryptorchidism is also characteristic. In other respects the phenotype is male (Fig. 5).

In most cases the uterus and tubes are discovered incidentally during surgery for cryptorchidism or an appendectomy. The gonads (testes) usually are located in the ovarian position. If these testes cannot be transposed into the scrotum, free testicular transplantation or gonadectomy and subse-

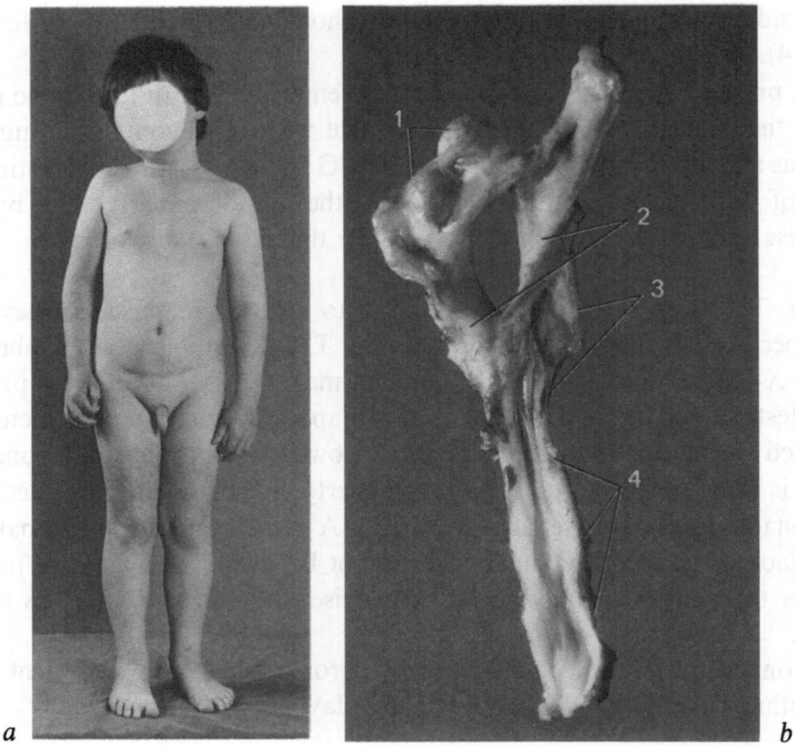

Fig. 5. (a) Boy with persistent müllerian ducts; (b) surgical specimen with uterus (3), *tubes* (2), *vagina* (4), *and testes* (1) *in the ovarian position*

quent androgen replacement should be considered. Because the situation is almost always unexpected, it is best to terminate the operation and seek consultation with the parents, endocrinologist and geneticist, so that a definitive plan of treatment can be made.

Congenital Anorchism

Occasionally boys are seen who have completely normal or mildly hypoplastic male external genitalia but have no palpable testes. Generally a normal male karyotype is present. Differentiation must be made in these cases between abdominal cryptorchidism and anorchism. Because the phenotype is male, functional testicular tissue must have been present during embryonic life. However, even high surgical exploration fails to reveal the presence of testes in the anorchid patient. Often the ductus deferens terminates blindly. In most cases the cause of the postembryonic loss of the testes remains undiscovered. These boys develop a characteristic hypergonadotropic hypogonadism during puberty.

It is significant therapeutically that the HCG test will reliably differentiate anorchism from abdominal cryptorchidism at any age (Fig. 6). Surgery is no longer considered appropriate in patients who lack palpable testes and have a negative HCG test.

Testosterone replacement should begin with normal doses for the child's age as soon as hypergonadotropic LH values develop. This usually occurs when these boys are between 11 and 12 years of age.

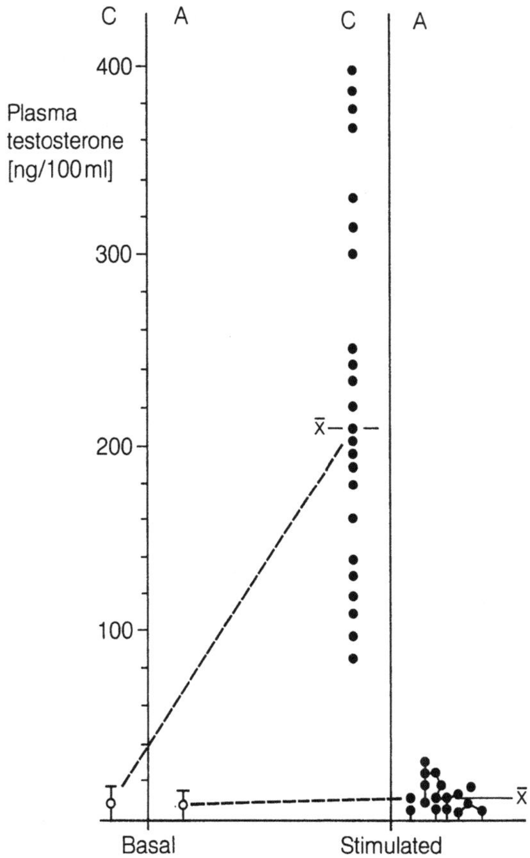

Fig. 6. Rise of plasma testosterone in the HCG test. C *Control group of boys with undescended testes;* A *prepubertal boys with anorchism*

Forms of Intersexuality Caused by Chromosomal Abnormalities

The possibility of an abnormality of the sex chromosomes (gonosomes) should be considered in every intersex patient whose hormonal status is unclear. Chromosome abnormalities are confirmed by karyography. The most common gonosomal aberrations, Klinefelter's syndrome (47 XXY), with a prevalence of 1:1000, and Ullrich-Turner syndrome (45 XO), with a prevalence of 1:2500, are of no importance in this context, because they are not associated with ambiguous genitals.

The principal gonosomal aberration from the standpoint of intersexuality is 45 XO/46 XY mosaicism. Clinical manifestations range from the complete picture of Ullrich-Turner syndrome to the almost normal male, depending on the predominance of a particular cell line. The syndrome involves a mixed gonadal dysgenesis with a predisposition to gonadoblastoma, which justifies the recommendation for early bilateral gonadectomy. The sex of rearing is decided by the patient's anatomy and his previous gender role. Following gonadectomy, replacement with testosterone or an estrogen/progestin product, depending on the assigned sex, is instituted at the age of puberty. Even when the phenotype is essentially male, a large rudimentary vagina can usually be demonstrated by urethrocystogenitography (Fig. 7). To date we have seen no reason why even a large rudimentary vagina cannot be left alone in patients with a male phenotype who have had a gonadectomy and are receiving testosterone replacement. Failure to remove an ovary or ovotestis will result in urethral menstrual bleeding.

Other typical gonosomal aberrations with intersexuality are the 46 XX/46 XY and 46 XX/47 XXY mosaicisms. Most of these cases involve true hermaphroditism, characterized by the coexistence of both testicular and ovarian tissue, either in the form of ovotestes or a testis on one side and an ovary on the other. A rudimentary vagina is generally present. An ovotestis or a gonad opposite to the patient's assigned sex should be removed before puberty. In asymmetrical mixed gonadal dysgenesis with a chromosomal mosaic the attempt to preserve a gonad is not advised owing to the risk of gonadoblastoma.

Fig. 7. (a) Child, reared as female, with 45 XO/46 XY chromosomal mosaic; (b) ambiguous external genitalia; (c) surgical specimen with testis (1) *and uterine tube* (2)*; (d) cystourethrogenitogram showing a large rudimentary vagina; urinary bladder* (1)*; proximal urethra* (2)*; vagina* (3)*; sinus urogenitalis communis* (4). *(Department of Radiology, Munich University Pediatric Clinic, Dr. Fendel, Director)*

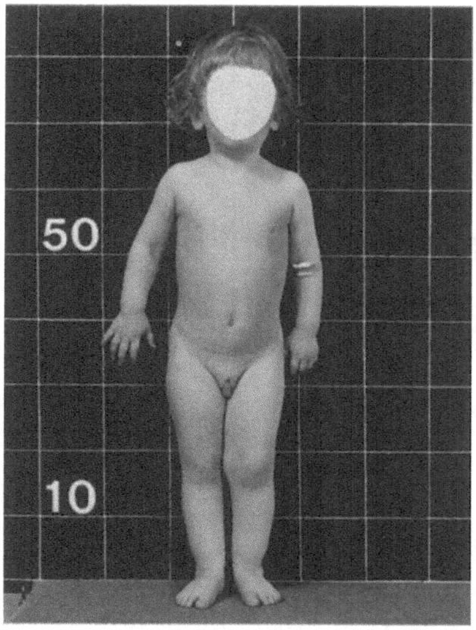

a

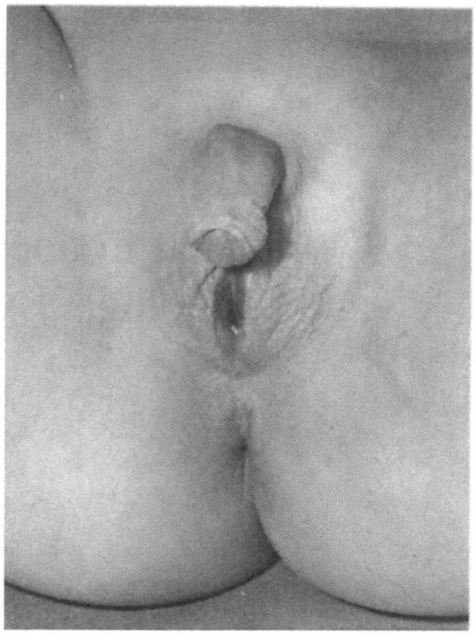

b

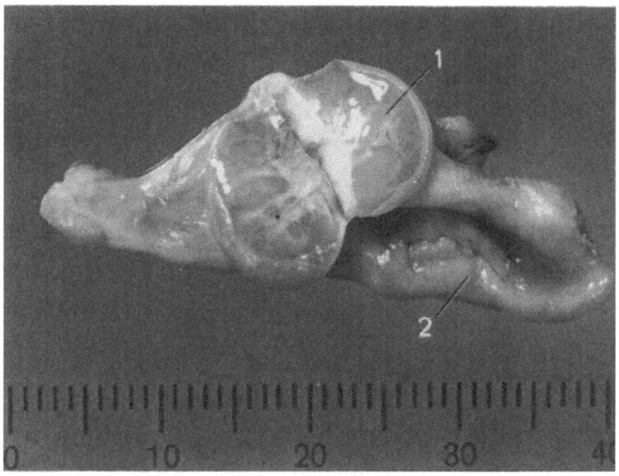

c

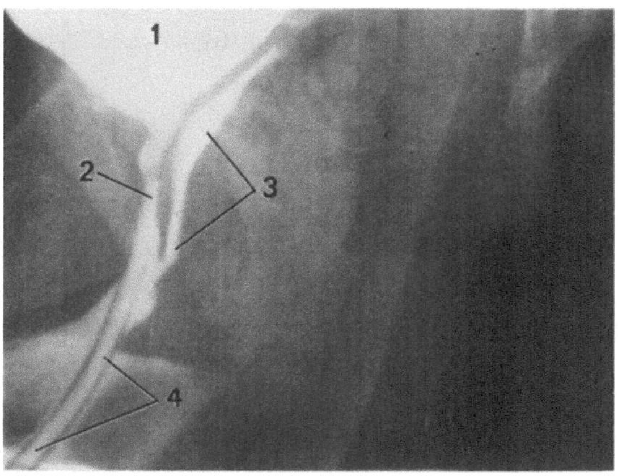

d

Principal Endocrinologic, Genetic, and Radiologic Examination Methods

HCG Test

This investigation tests the body's ability to form normal amounts of testosterone. It can be done at any age. The main role of the HCG test (e.g., Predalon, Primogonyl, Pregnesin) is to differentiate between bilateral anorchism and abdominal cryptorchidism. It is also used to detect disturbances of testosterone biosynthesis in prepubertal children.

Procedure
Day 1: 5 ml Heparinized plasma is drawn for basal testosterone. Then 5000 IU HCG is administered i.m. (3000 IU i.m. for infants).
Day 2: Another 5 ml heparinized plasma is drawn (stimulated value).

Evaluation. The true testosterone level of prepubertal boys is approximately 10 ng/dl. In these cases the specimen should be purified by one chromatographic run prior to radioimmunoassay. Following HCG, the plasma testosterone normally rises to an average of 210 ng/dl (90–400 ng/dl) in prepuberty. In anorchism, no rise is elicited (Fig. 6).

HMG Test

The HMG test is used to demonstrate normal ovarian endocrine function. The test is not as reliable or as widely used as the HCG test. Its main role is in confirming pure gonadal dysgenesis.

Procedure

Day 1: Heparinized blood is drawn to determine the basal estradiol. Then 75 IU/day HMG is administered i.m. on 3 consecutive days.

Day 4: Heparinized blood is drawn to determine the stimulated estradiol.

Evaluation. A significant rise of plasma estradiol proves the existence of ovarian tissue with adequate endocrine function.

Karyography

It is best to draw the necessary heparinized blood at the site of the cell culture. But a culture can also be prepared from heparinized blood that has been sterilely drawn and rushed to the laboratory. The test must be scheduled beforehand with the genetic facility to avoid loss of time.

Simple determination of the cell chromatin from leukocytes, buccal epithelium, or hair follicles is not sufficient for the present purposes.

Individual cell lines in chromosome mosaics often are present in very small numbers, and so large numbers of mitoses must be examined before they are detected. In some circumstances the blood culture should be supplemented by a fibroblast culture prepared from a skin biopsy. Such tests are extremely time-consuming and require that the patient be notified of the result at a later date.

Urethrocystogenitography

The demonstration of a rudimentary vagina with contrast radiographs is indicated in all patients with intersexual genitals. The result will influence the assigned sex of rearing and the nature of the surgical procedure, and it may have a bearing on differential diagnosis. Care must be taken in interpreting the urethrocystogenitogram, for failure to demonstrate a vagina does not disprove its existence! The apparent absence of a vagina may be due to adhesions of the introitus or to an error in technique. The procedure should be done by an examiner who is familiar with the patient's age group and with the technique. As the procedure may be alarming to many children, we usually administer a short-acting general anesthetic. It is important that the gonads be placed directly in the cone of the x-ray beam during the examination.

Part 2
Surgical Measures for the Correction of Intersexual Genitalia and Female Genital Malformations

General Guidelines Regarding the Optimum Timing of Corrective Surgery and Studies Necessary for Preoperative Planning

Prader (1954) has divided the degrees of malformation of intersexual genitalia into five grades ranging from the purely female type to the purely male type. Intersexual genitals can vary greatly in their anatomy, and in extreme cases the external morphology may be the opposite of the patient's chromosomal sex (Fig. 1).

A surgical classification of intersexual genitals is presented in Table 1. In true hermaphroditism the internal genitalia may consists of one testis and one ovary, one testis or ovary in association with one ovotestis, or two ovotestes. In male pseudohermaphroditism the gonads are always testes, and in female pseudohermaphroditism they are always ovaries. However, the external genitalia of these patients can show a variety of forms, ranging from purely female to purely male.

Female pseudohermaphroditism is by far the most prevalent type, and the adrenogenital syndrome (CAH) is its principal cause. Female intersex is also seen in association with virilizing adrenocortical tumors and in children whose mothers took hormones or had hormone-secreting neoplasms during pregnancy.

Table 1. Classification of intersexual genitalia. (Adapted from Hienz 1969)

	True hermaphroditism	Pseudohermaphroditism	
		Male	Female
Internal genitalia	Testis + ovary Testis or ovary + ovotestis Ovotestis + ovotestis	Testis	Ovary
External genitalia	Ambiguous from pure male to pure female		

Whenever intersexuality is suspected, it is imperative that a chromosomal analysis be performed. In the case of mosaicism, the analysis should be done twice to eliminate any chance of error. This is important, because in such cases the gonads are highly susceptible to malignant change, and gonadectomy is imperative. Other necessary investigations include electrolyte status, gonadotropin and steroid assays, genitography, and possibly ultrasonography to visualize the internal genitalia. Genitograms are crucial to preoperative planning, as they guide the surgeon is selecting the most suitable procedure.

The timing of corrective surgery for intersexual genitals is a critical matter. The goal of all therapeutic efforts is to enable the intersexual patient to live a normal life both physically and psychologically.

From the standpoint of personality development, it is essential that the child acquire a sexual identity at an early age. According to Hassenstein (quoted in Hemminger 1982), there are five main forces which shape the acquistion of sexual identity (Fig. 8). These are the chromosomal sex, the morphological sex, the sex of rearing, biologically based sex-specific behav-

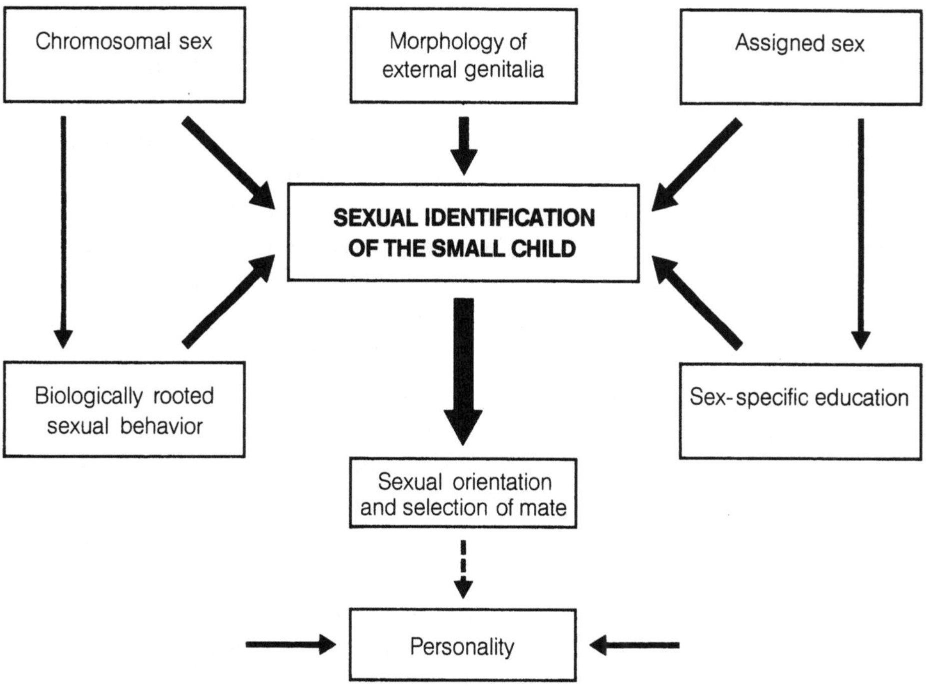

Fig. 8. The factors governing human sexual differentiation. (Adapted from Hassenstein, quoted in Hemminger 1982)

ioral tendencies, and sex-specific education. All these forces, which interact to some degree, cause the child to acquire a sexual identity between the ages of 2 and 3. This sexual identification will determine the child's later sexual orientation and the selection of a mate, and according to Hassenstein, will shape a range of aspects, from the individual's psychosocial gender role to his sexuality, becoming an integral part of the way in which he views humanity and the world.

It is possible to influence three important factors in the sexual identification of the small child. First, the morphology of the external genitalia can be altered by surgical means. Second, the child's registered sex can be changed on the basis of medical certification. Third, one can influence the sex-specific education of the child, which is chiefly a parental responsibility. Because the correct sexual identification of the small child has a profound impact on subsequent personality development, necessary corrections should be undertaken as soon as possible. We share the opinion of the Zurich pediatric endocrinologist Prader that unconfused, sex-specific rearing of the small child by parents can take place only if the child's external genitalia conform to its sexual identity. In other words, it is difficult to raise a child as a boy when the child's external genitals are obviously female, and vice versa.

Thus, it is imperative that the surgical correction of ambiguous genitalia be undertaken at the earliest possible age, and certainly before a sexual identity is acquired, i.e., before the child's second birthday.

What approach should be taken in children who have been pronounced to be one sex on the basis of their external genitalia, but whose chromosomal sex is different? These are cases in which three of the five factors shown in Fig. 8 are operating incorrectly. We feel that the parents of these children should be allowed to make a decision without pressure from the physician. The doctor should advise the parents but should not suggest the direction of their decision. The pediatric surgeon, aided by the pediatrician and possibly a psychologist, should make it clear to the parents that, whatever decision is reached, he will be able to reconstruct the external genitalia along male or female lines, as required. This is stated only to aid the parents in making their decision. From a medical standpoint, the most appropriate solution would be a surgical correction that conforms to the child's chromosomal sex. However, a complete change of sex always represents a serious social problem for the patient and the family. We have seen children with adrenogenital syndrome and external genitalia of Prader type V who were reared as males for several years before their true chromosomal sex was discovered and whose parents did not desire a sex reversal. In these cases the gonads were removed, hormonal replacement was instituted at a later age, and the patients went on to have an undisturbed childhood and puberty. In addition, we have seen cases of male hermaphroditism with Prader type IV external genitalia and a very small phallus which prompted pediatricians and psychologists to advise that the child be reared as a girl and that the genitalia be reconstructed accordingly. This recommendation conflicted with the wishes of the parents, and subsequently we were able to construct a satisfactory male organ capable of normal erection and coitus.

In true hermaphroditism it is imperative that the gonads be removed, regardless of whether a masculinizing or feminizing operation is contemplated. It is impossible to tell from the external appearance of a gonad whether it is an ovary, a testis, or an ovotestis. Hormonal replacement is then instituted in acordance with the selected sex of rearing.

Correction of Clitoral Hypertrophy and Urogenital Sinus with Low Vaginal Entry

When the external genitalia are to be reconstructed along female lines, the first step is to determine the level at which the vagina enters the urogenital sinus. Usually this can be assessed by means of genitography (Fig. 7d), but if this is not sufficient endoscopy (uteroscopy) will be required. It must be determined whether the correction can be effected by a simple vaginoplasty or whether the vagina will have to be detached from the urogenital sinus and pulled through to the perineum. The surgical approach differs for each procedure. If preoperative studies indicate a low vaginal entry, but a vaginal orifice is not found at operation, the operation should be terminated, the urogenital sinus closed, and the previously mobilized skin flap sutured back into place. A vaginal pullthrough operation can then be performed about 6 months later (see p. 50).

Regardless of whether the vagina enters high or low, we prefer to correct the hypertrophied clitoris and urogenital sinus in a single operation. It would be possible to perform both procedures separately, but it is better to avoid a second operation if at all possible, and the patients tolerate the complete revision very well.

Numerous surgical techniques are available for correction of the hypertrophied clitoris and urogenital sinus. While amputation of the enlarged clitoris was routinely practiced before the work of Stephan (1966) was published, for the past 2 decades surgeons have attempted either to spare the clitoris in its entirety or to resect the shaft and leave the glans intact. The main proponents of the resection method are Marberger et al. (1975) and Engert (1983). Stephan showed in the 1950s that the clitoral shaft could be buckled with plicating sutures and recessed behind the pubic symphysis in such a way that the glans is adequately concealed by the labia during lying, standing, and sitting. Bolkenius and Daum (1977) then showed how "labia minora" could be made from the skin of the prepuce. Flach (1977) dissects a large skin flap from the prepuce and shaft and advances it into the operative area of the perineum, in this way creating "skin bulges" which conceal the glans after recession of the shaft.

Various techniques are also available for opening the urogenital sinus, all of which are based on the original suggestion of Stephan to mobilize an inverted U-shaped flap of perineal skin, open the urogenital sinus, and suture the anally based flap to the posterior wall of the opened vagina.

Our procedure, which we have used successfully in more than 140 patients, is as follows (Fig. 9): The patient is placed in the lithotomy position with thighs fully abducted. The area is draped in such a way that the rectum is accessible for palpation (especially useful in low forms of urogenital sinus). A probe is inserted into the urogenital sinus to locate the lowest point of the sinus below the perineal skin, just before the sinus and urethra curve away from the perineum toward the bladder. This point is marked to indicate the base of an M-shaped, anally based perineal skin flap, which is also outlined with a marker. The M-shaped flap should extend about two-thirds of the distance from the marked low point of the urogenital sinus to the sinus opening (Fig. 9a). The flap is dissected free, and stay sutures are placed through its cranial corners. Two additional stay sutures (6-O Ethibond) are placed to the right and left of the sinus opening, and the urogenital sinus is opened with several snips of the scissors. When the urethral orifice is identified a Foley catheter is passed into the bladder. Now the back wall of the vagina is defined, and the introitus is opened until an adequate width is achieved. The previously mobilized M-shaped perineal skin flap is sutured with 5-0 or 6-0 Vicryl to the posterior commissure of the introitus. The opened wall of the urogenital sinus is sutured to the perineal skin using the same material. The vagina is tamponaded with rolled strips of tulle (Sofratull) for 4 days postoperatively, and bucrylate adhesive is applied to the wound edges.

To correct the hypertrophied clitoris, we first place a stay suture through the glans and then incise the dorsal shaft skin on the midline from the mons pubis to the base of the glans, continuing the incision around the glans in semicircular fashion 1 mm from the coronal sulcus. The skin is mobilized from the dorsal and lateral aspects of the shaft, and the preputial skin is unfurled to make a pair of triangular flaps. Exposure of the clitoral shaft is then continued in the direction of the symphysis, dissecting back to the division of the corpora and exposing both crura for a length of 1–1.5 cm. Next the caudodorsal portion of the pubic symphysis is dissected free. Plication of the clitoral shaft is effected in two stages. First, nonabsorbable sutures are run from each crus to the middle of the shaft and tied. Then additional plicating sutures are placed from the proximal third of the shaft to within a short distance of the glans. These sutures (3-0 or 4-0 Ethiflex) are also tied. The ends are left long, and they are passed through the periosteum of the symphysis with a small periosteal needle and tied. The effect of this procedure is two-fold: The clitoral shaft is shortened by the plication, and the clitoris is recessed behind the symphysis.

The triangular skin flaps that were formed by unfolding the prepuce and which extend laterally to the right and left of the glans are engaged at their apices with stay sutures and then sutured to themselves and later to the preputial remnant on the coronal sulcus in such a way that the bases of the flaps, which are to form the labia minora, come to lie craniolateral to the glans. This will ensure complete coverage of the glans by the labia. Two layers of subcutaneous sutures (6-0 or 5-0 Vicryl) are placed over the phallus shaft and symphysis, and the skin is closed with the same material. Bucrylate is applied to the wound.

The Foley catheter is left in place for one week, and vaginal tamponade is maintained for four days.

In children who are not yet toilet trained, the legs should be extended vertically (Fig. 10), as for a femoral fracture, to keep feces away from the wound area. This position is maintained until satisfactory wound healing has occurred.

The labia minora formed from the prepuce will occasionally vary in size. However, a secondary correction, which can be done as an outpatient procedure, should be undertaken no sooner than 6 months after the primary operation. During subsequent follow-ups it is necessary to confirm that the vaginal introitus is not contracting, but is growing with the patient. This is always the case in patients with AGS who are receiving regular corticoid therapy, and we have found that the newly formed vagina tends to grow satisfactorily in other patients as well. We initially check for stenosis under general anesthesia, and then on subsequent visits we use Hegar dilators without anesthesia. This examination is done every 6 months for the first 3–4 years and thereafter at yearly intervals until the child is grown.

Fig. 9a. Patient with urogenital sinus and clitoral hypertrophy. A metal sound is introduced into the urogenital sinus to locate the lowest part of the sinus close to the perineal skin. That point (visible as a bulge at the probe tip) marks the base of an M-shaped skin flap, which is outlined with a marker and incised

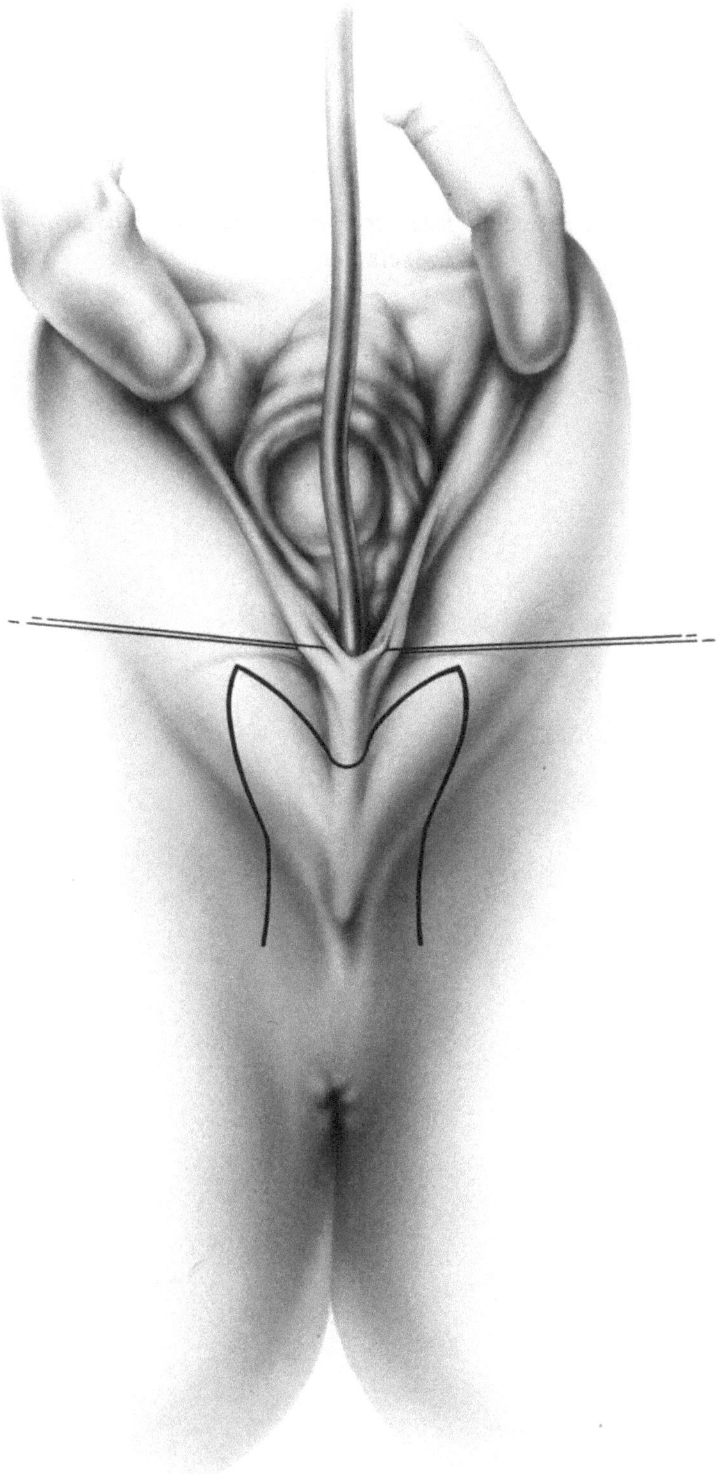

Fig. 9b. The flap is dissected free, and the urogenital sinus is opened with scissors

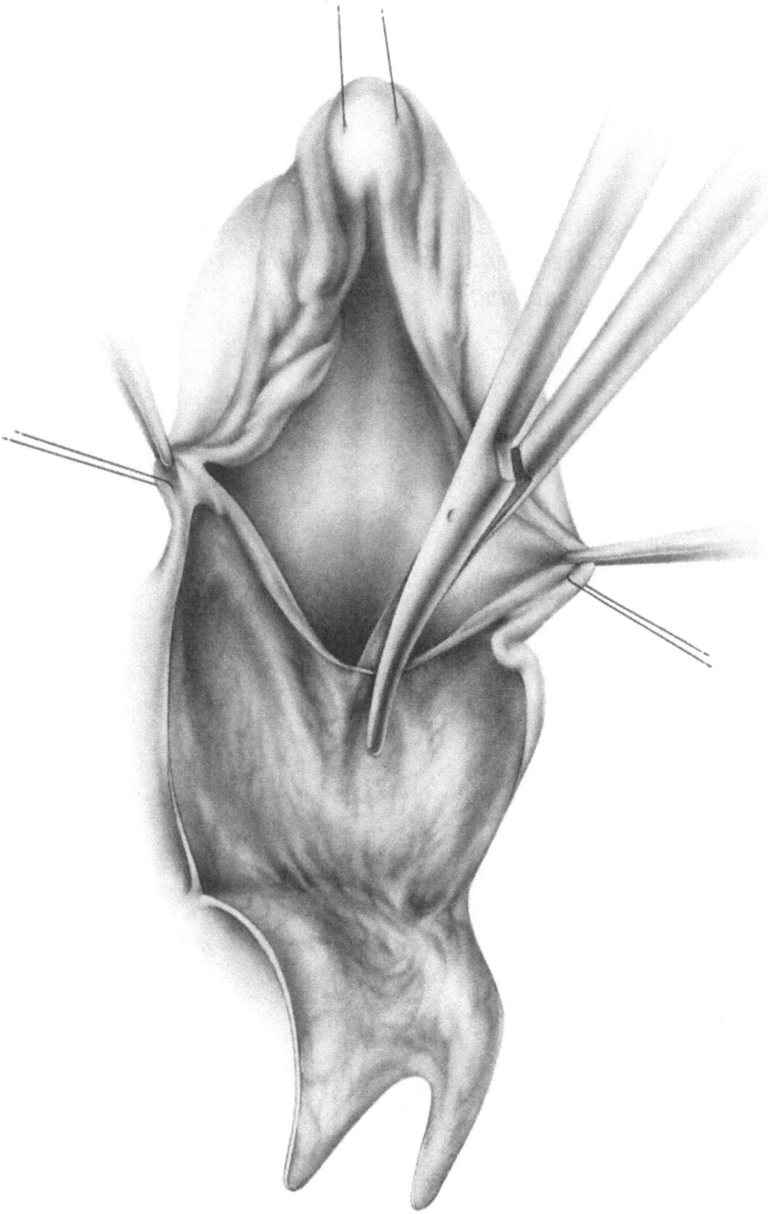

Fig. 9c. The flap is sutured to the posterior vaginal commissure, the lateral ends being sutured to the vagina as far cranially as possible. The urethra and bladder are catheterized

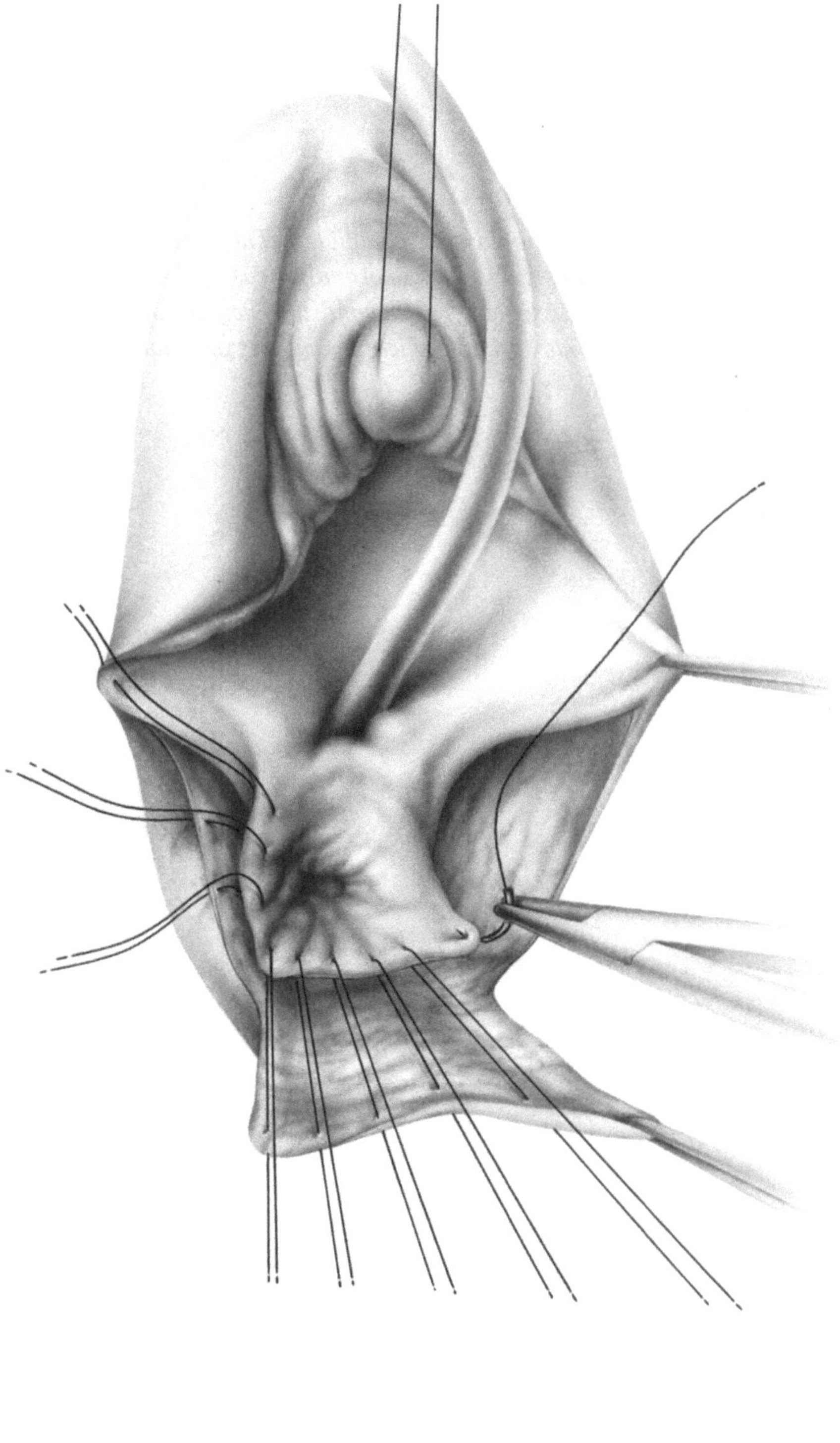

Fig. 9d. Top left *The flap vaginoplasty is completed. The dorsal clitoroplasty incision extends from the mons pubis to the coronal sulcus of the glans.* Center *The shaft of the clitoris is dissected free beyond the division of the corpora cavernosa, and nonabsorbable plicating sutures are placed*

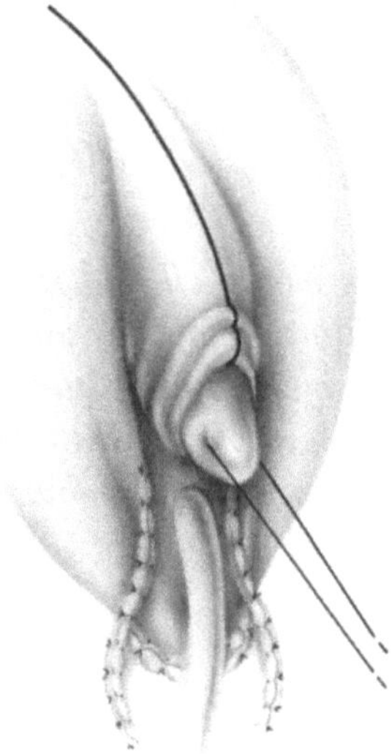

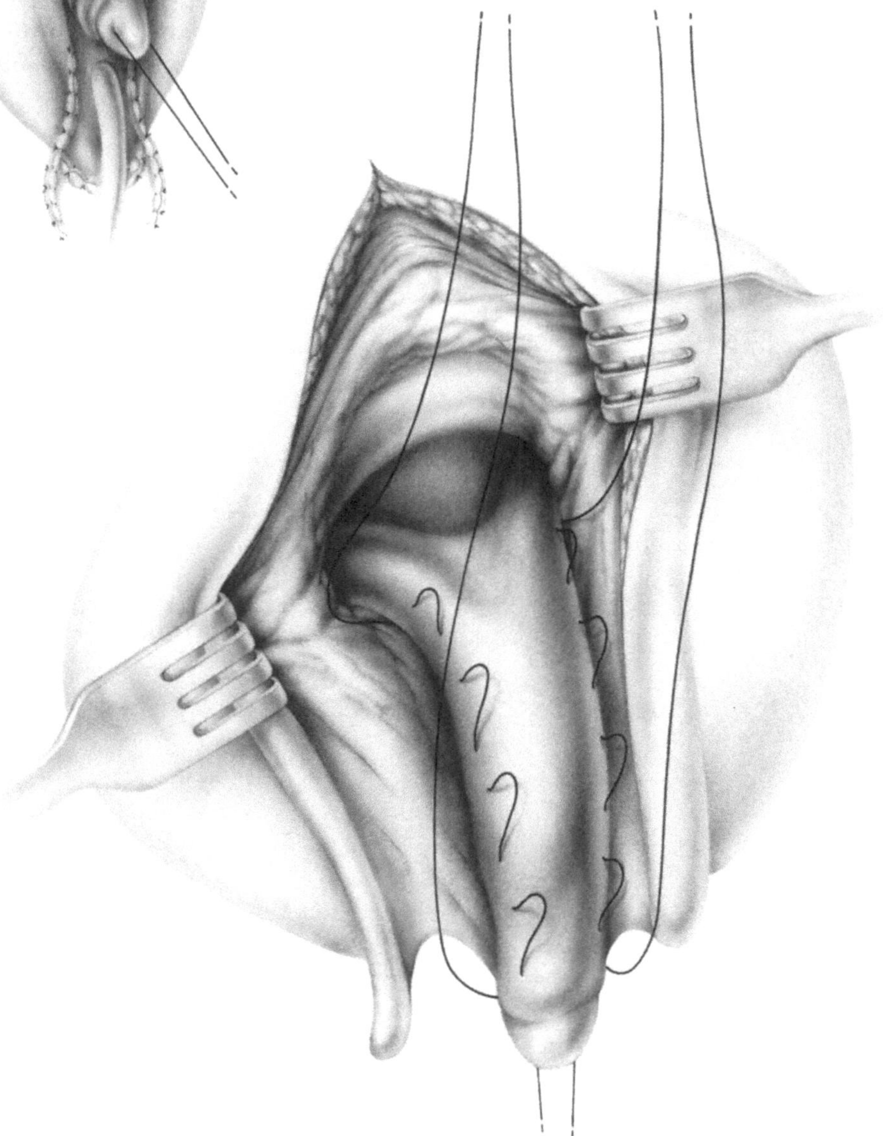

Fig. 9e. Top left *Lateral view of the plicating sutures in the clitoral shaft.* Top right *The plicating stitches are tied, and the clitoral shaft is sutured to the periosteum of the pubic symphysis.* Center *AP view of the situation at upper right. The clitoral shaft ist attached to the symphysis with two nonabsorbable sutures. Note the lateral, winglike flaps formed by the mobilized prepuce*

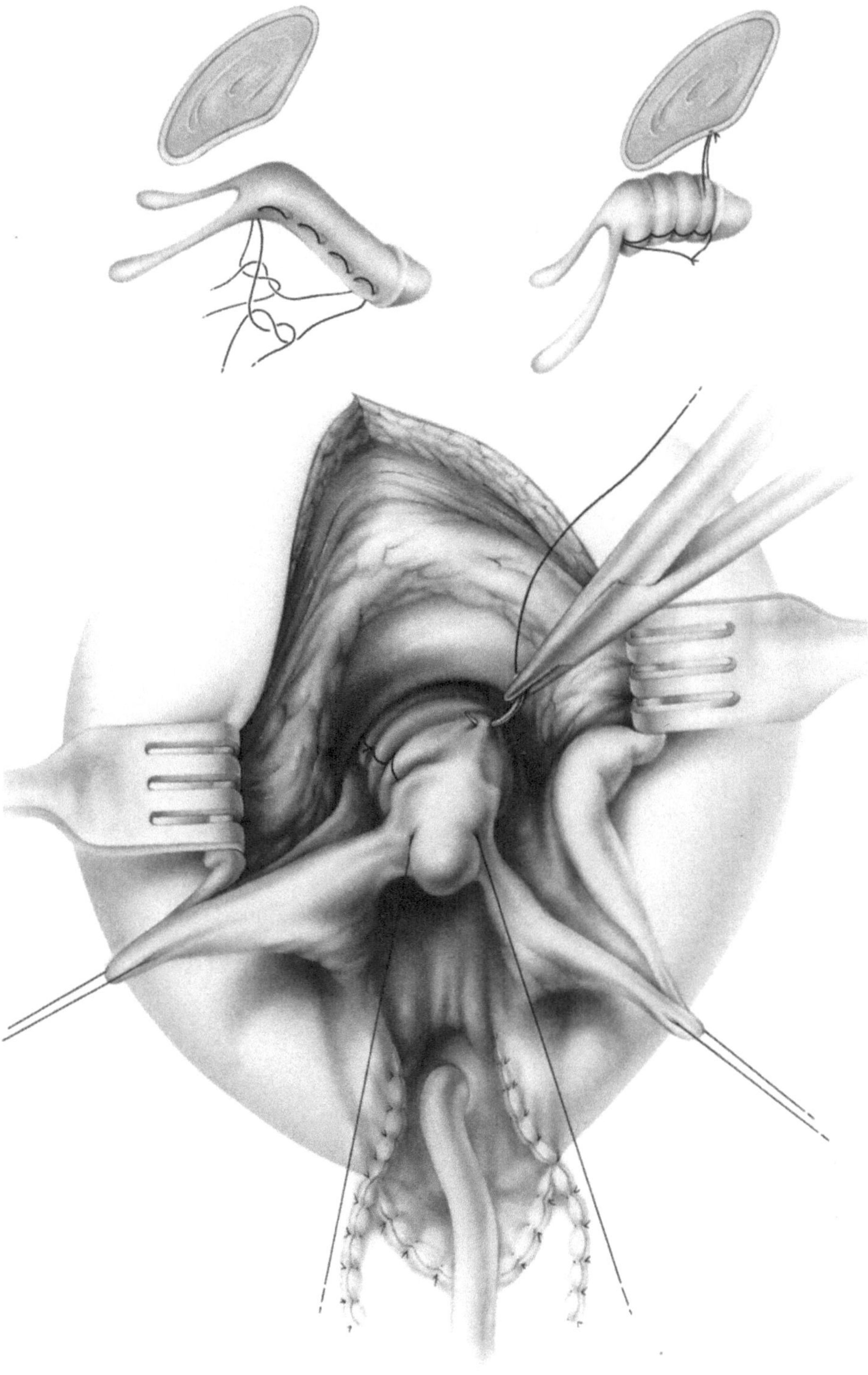

Fig. 9f. Labia minora are made from the prepuce by suturing the edges of each flap together and then to the glans in such a way that the glans is concealed

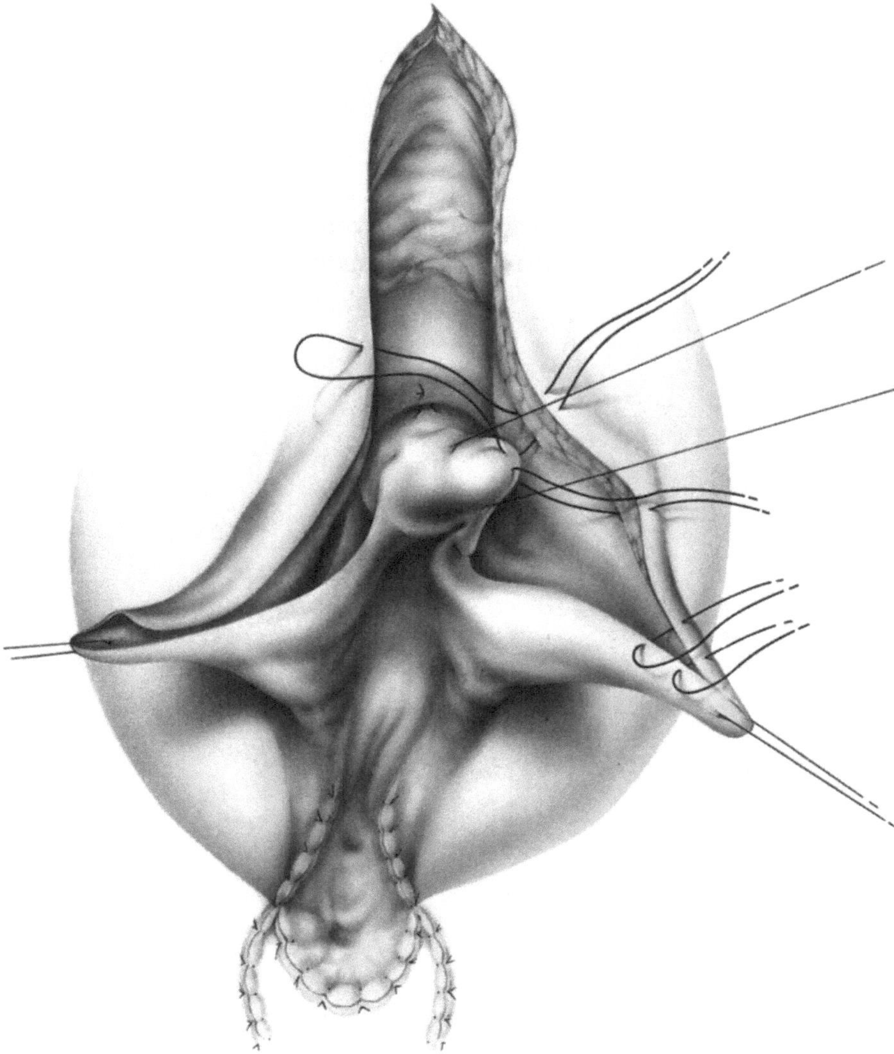

Fig. 9g. Postoperative appearance of the introitoplasty and clitoroplasty, showing the "labia minora" constructed from the prepuce

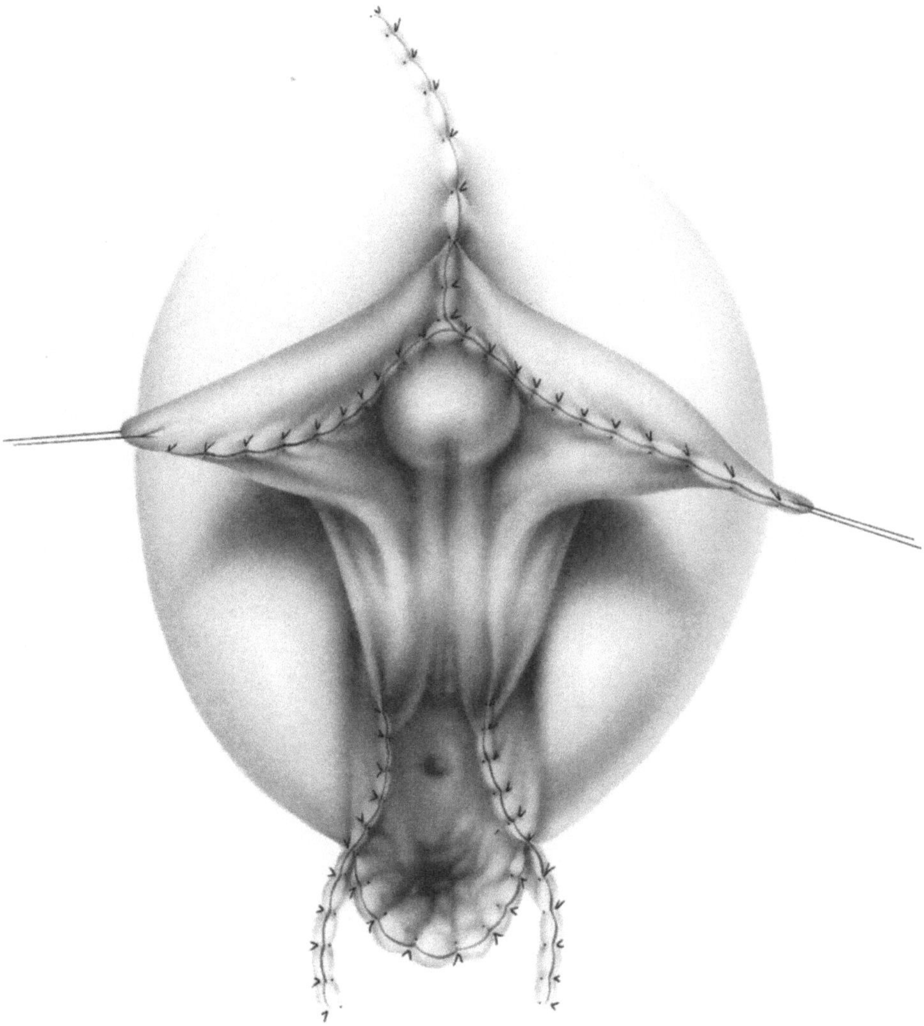

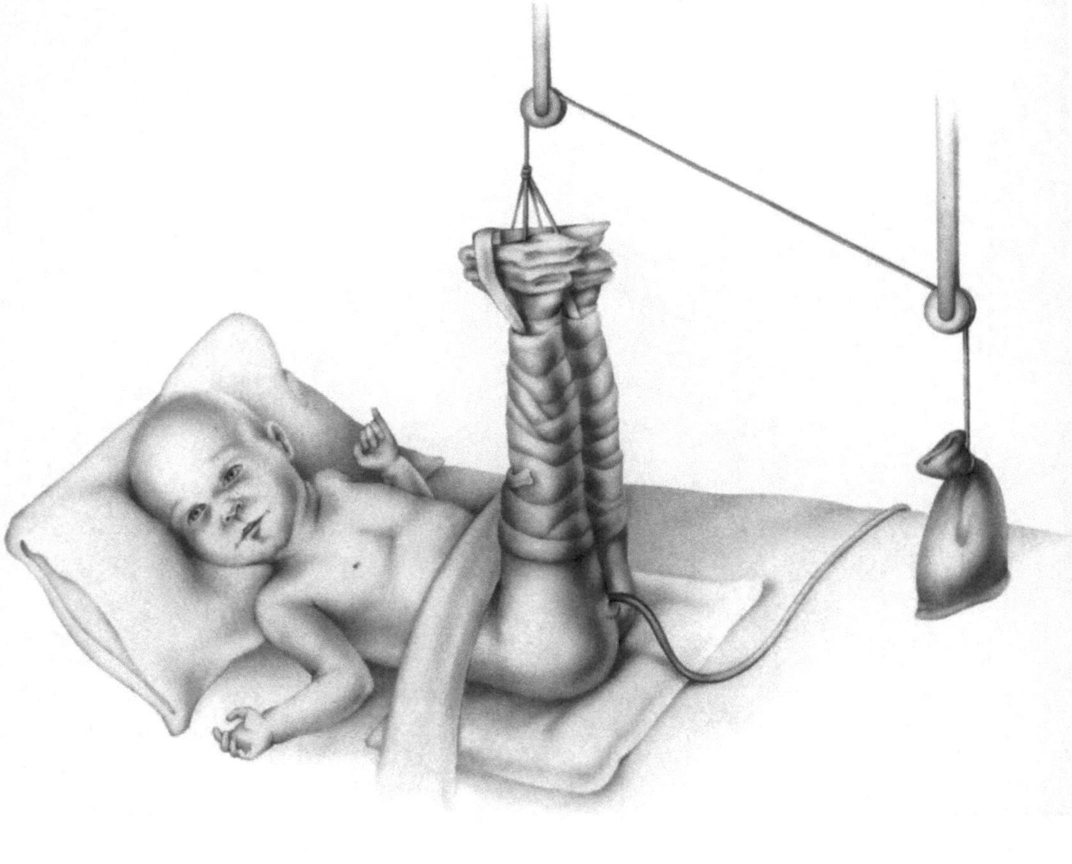

Fig. 10. Vertical extension of both legs, similar to the traction used for femoral fractures. The buttocks are suspended a handwidth above mattress to prevent fecal soiling of the wound region

Secondary Correction to Improve Glans Coverage

Formerly, when we did not use the prepuce to make labia minora, there were many instances where satisfactory glans coverage was not achieved. In these patients, as well as in cases where the labia minora plasty does not conceal the glans adequately, we recommend the following secondary correction (Fig. 11), which is based on a suggestion of Ansel and Rajfer (1981): A skin incision is made around the glans 10 mm from its base, the skin edges are dissected free on all sides, and the medial edges closest to the glans are joined together with inverting sutures so as to conceal the glans. Then the outer skin edges are approximated with vertical mattress sutures (5-0 or 6-0 Vicryl). With this technique the glans is concealed but can still be demonstrated. The patient need not be hospitalized.

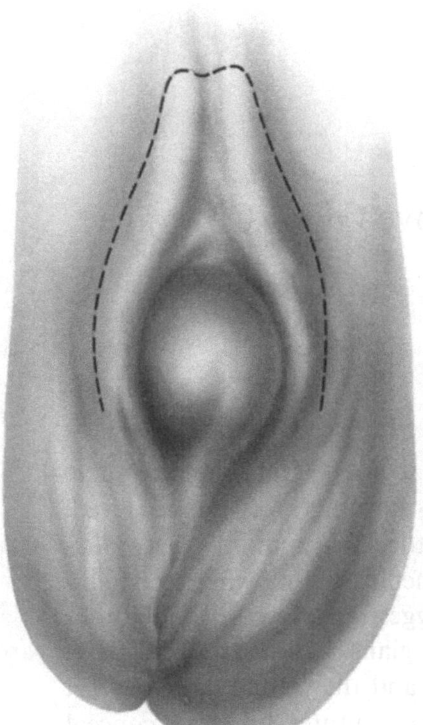

a

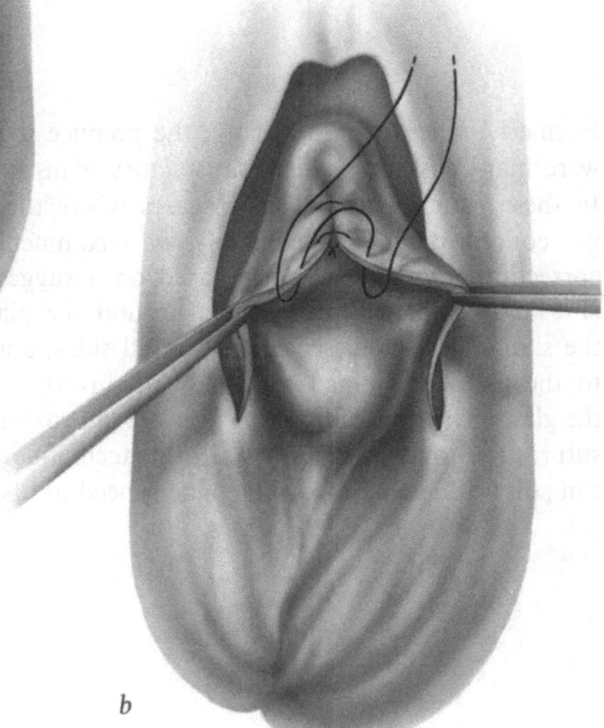

b

Fig. 11a–d. Secondary operation to correct inadequate glans coverage by the labia minora or majora

Fig. 11a. A labial incision is made around the glans (about 1–1.5 cm from the clitoris), and the wound edges are mobilized

Fig. 11b. The medial edges are joined with inverting sutures

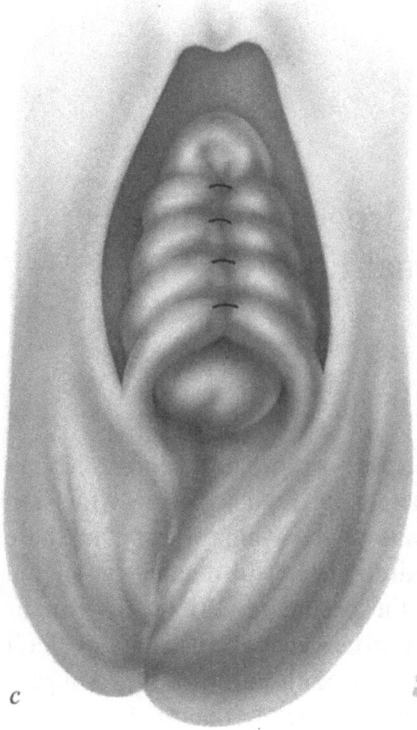

c

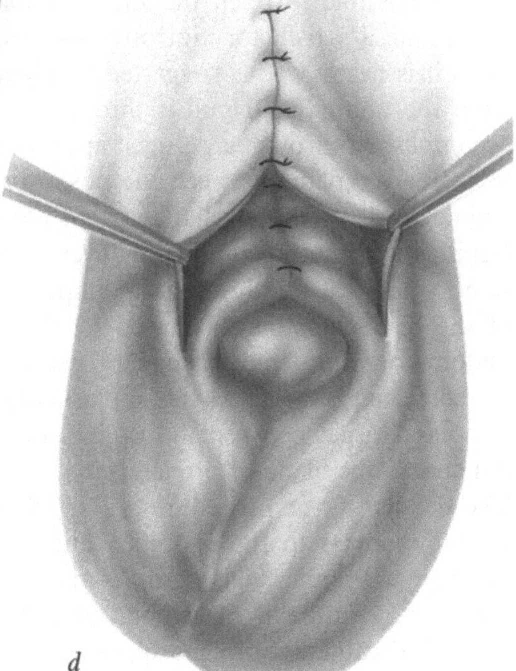

d

Fig. 11c. Appearance of the sutured medial skin flaps.

Fig. 11d. The lateral skin edges are approximated, leaving about one-quarter of the glans visible. This portion will be satisfactorily concealed by the labia majora

Surgical Correction of Urogenital Sinus with High Vaginal Entry

If the vagina enters the urogenital sinus close to the bladder neck, it may not be possible to open the sinus completely through a perineal incision and create a satisfactory introitus by means of flap vaginoplasty. In these cases it is necessary, as suggested by Hendren (1980), to detach the vagina from the urethra and pull it through to the perineum. While this can be accomplished through a perineal approach, it becomes increasingly difficult to define the plane between the posterior wall of the urethra and anterior vaginal wall as the level of vaginal entry approaches the bladder. Since significant urinary incontinence developed in one of our patients who underwent a perineal pullthrough vaginoplasty, presumably because of a lesion of the bladder sphincter caused by the dissection, we have developed an abdominoperineal pullthrough procedure that is similar to the procedure for correcting subtotal vaginal aplasia described below. With this technique it is easy to get between the vagina, urethra, and bladder without risking damage to the bladder sphincter.

The details of our procedure are as follows (Fig. 12): The field is draped to allow access to the abdomen and perineum. The abdomen is entered through a Pfannenstiel incision, and the bowel is retracted cranially. A strong stay suture is placed through the uterus, after which dissection is continued caudally into the space between the bladder and uterus and between the rectum and vagina. The initial part of this dissection is done with a scalpel, but the major portion is done bluntly. The junction of the vagina and urogenital sinus is easily demonstrated. Following this exposure, the operation is continued through a perineal approach. The proposed vaginal pullthrough site on the perineum is identified, and two laterally based skin flaps, each 1–1.5 cm wide and 3–4 cm long (depending on the size of the child), are mobilized at that location. Later these skin flaps will be swung into the vagina and anastomosed to it. The operator now dissects cranially through the perineal incision, aided by a Foley catheter passed through the urethra and a finger inserted into the rectum. The deepest point of the abdominal dissection is easily reached and should be marked by means of a dissecting patty introduced into the abdomen by an assistant. This patty can be felt by the operator dissecting from the perineum.

The abdominal and perineal fields having been joined, a rubber sling is passed around the vagina, grasped from the perineum and pulled caudally until the confluence of the vagina and urogenital sinus is visualized. Two stay sutures are placed through the vagina, and the vaginal attachment is transected from the urogenital sinus in a stepwise fashion while simultaneously the sinus is closed (5-0 or 6-0 Vicryl); this now serves as the urethra. The stay sutures are used to pull the vaginal orifice down to the mobilized perineal skin flaps, to which it is anastomosed with 6-0 or 7-0 Vicryl. Usually it is possible to join the perineal skin flaps and the vagina in such a way that complete perineal wound coverage is obtained. A drain is then inserted into the vagina to serve as a stent, where it remains until wound closure is complete, i.e., the wound bed is completely epithelialized. A suction drain is also inserted through a separate perineal stab incision. Meanwhile the abdominal team has closed the peritoneum and abdominal incision. If the patient is not toilet trained the legs are extended vertically. The bladder catheter is left place for 14 days; withdrawal of the catheter is combined with a micturating cystourethrogram (MCU) to document healing of the urethra (sinus). Growth of the newly created vaginal introitus is checked periodically by the introduction of Hegar dilators.

If the clitoris is hypertrophied, as is usually the case, it is also corrected during the same session using the technique described under "Correction of Clitoral Hypertrophy and Urogenital Sinus with Low Vaginal Entry."

Fig. 12a–i. Correction of urogenital sinus with a high vaginal entry

***Fig. 12a.** The abdomen is opened through a Pfannenstiel incision, and the vesicouterine pouch is reached by dissection. The uterus is either grasped with an Allis clamp or engaged with stay sutures, as is the urinary bladder. The peritoneum between the bladder and uterus is incised with a scalpel or scissors, and dissection is continued into the vesicouterine space*

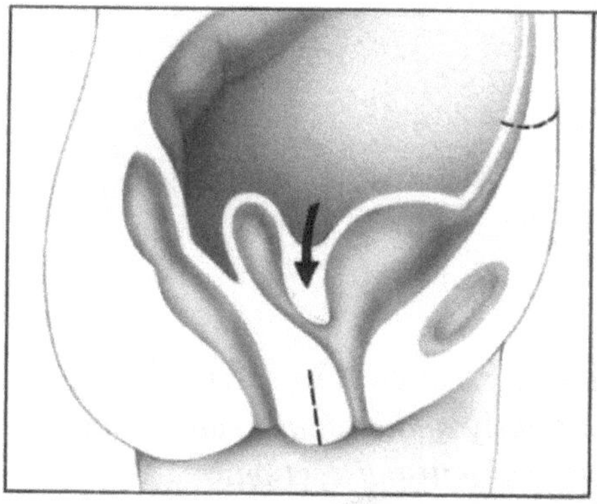

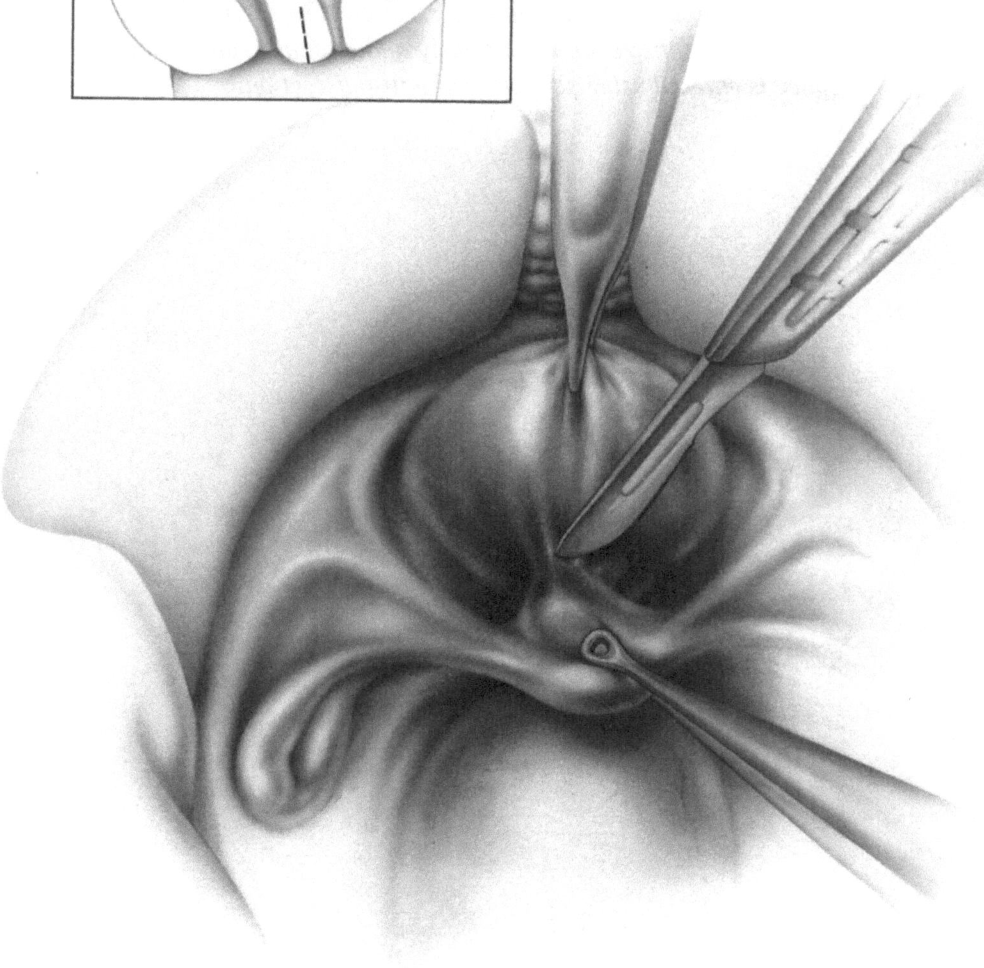

Fig. 12b. The pouch of Douglas is reached by dissection. The uterus is retracted anteriorly and caudally, the rectum posteriorly and cranially, and Douglas' space is entered using scissors and patty dissection

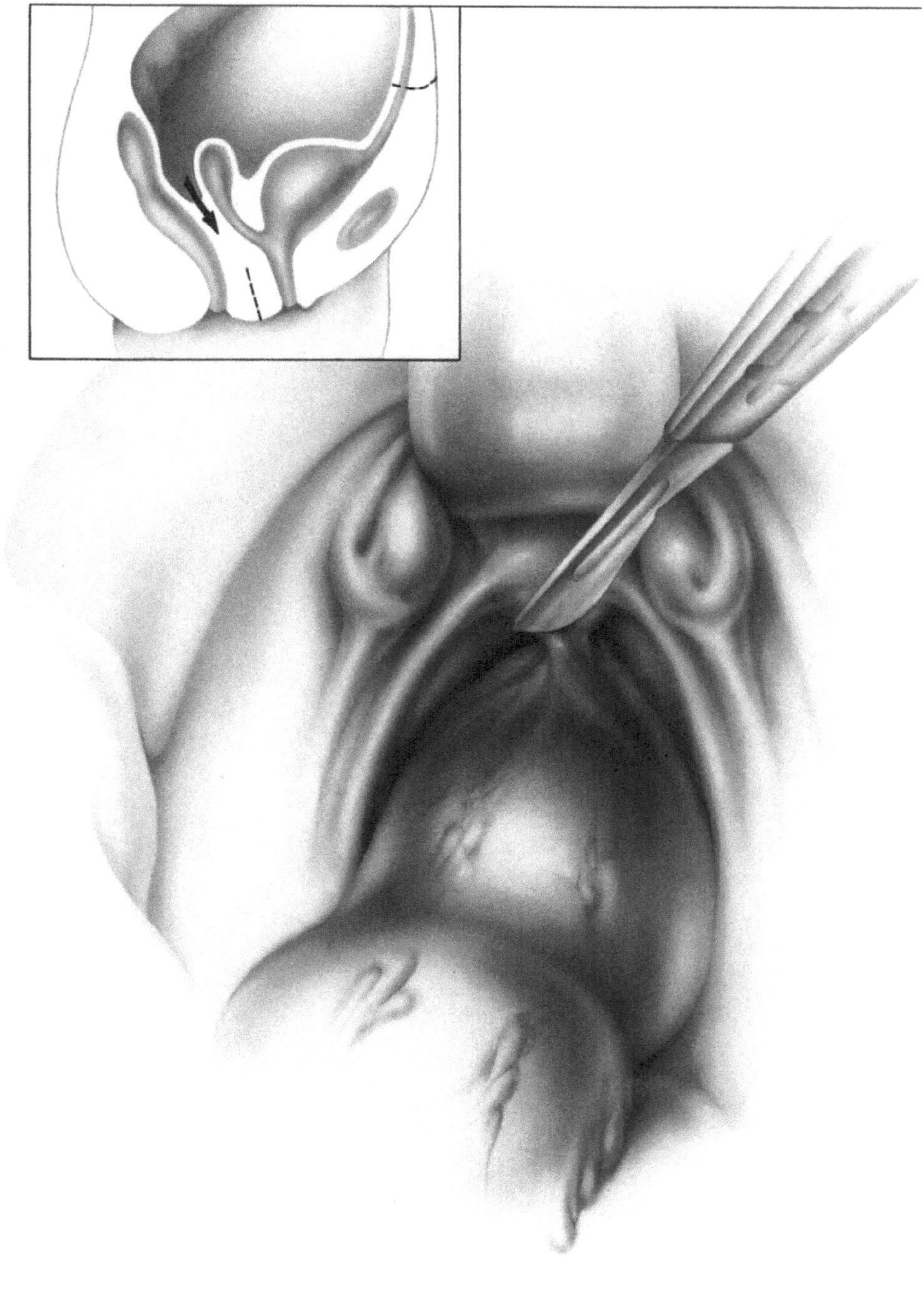

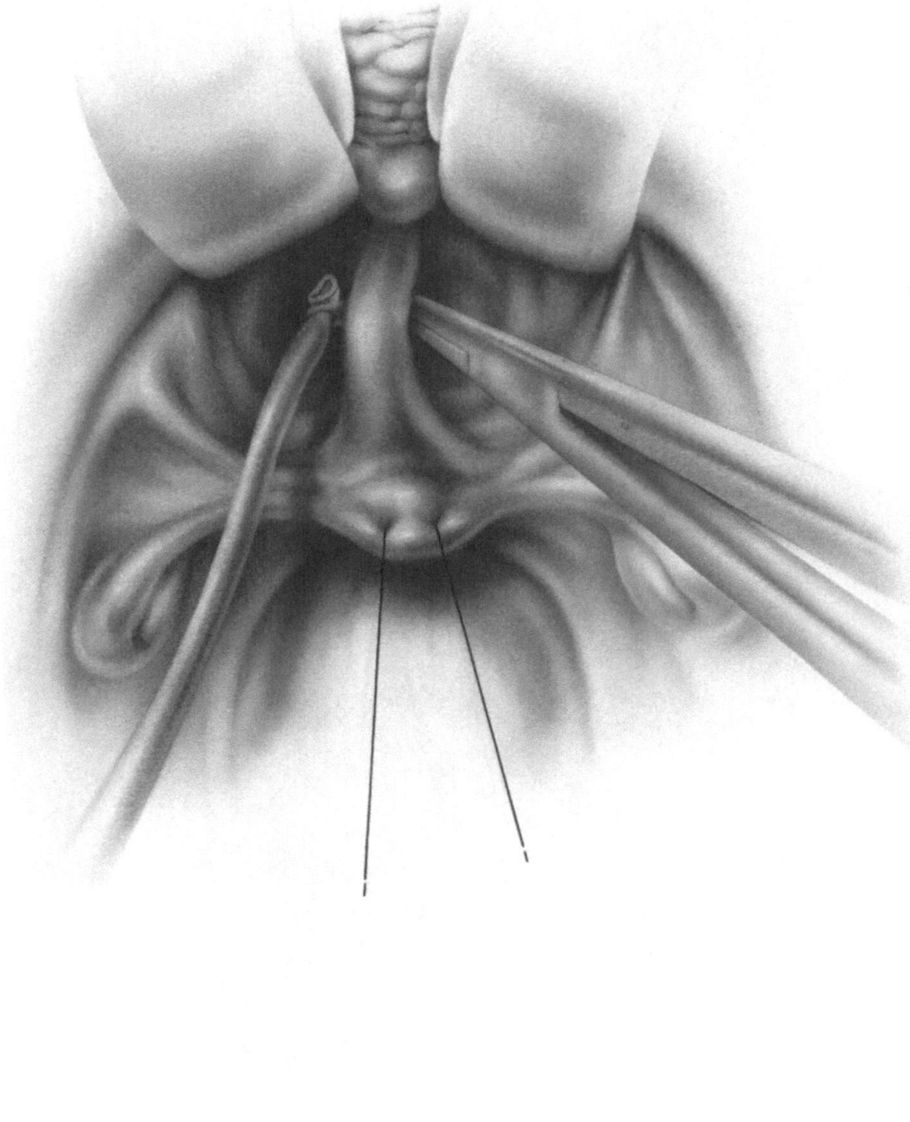

Fig. 12c. After the junction of the uterus and vagina has been exposed, a sling is passed around the upper part of the vagina with an Overholt clamp so that cranial tension can be placed on the vagina

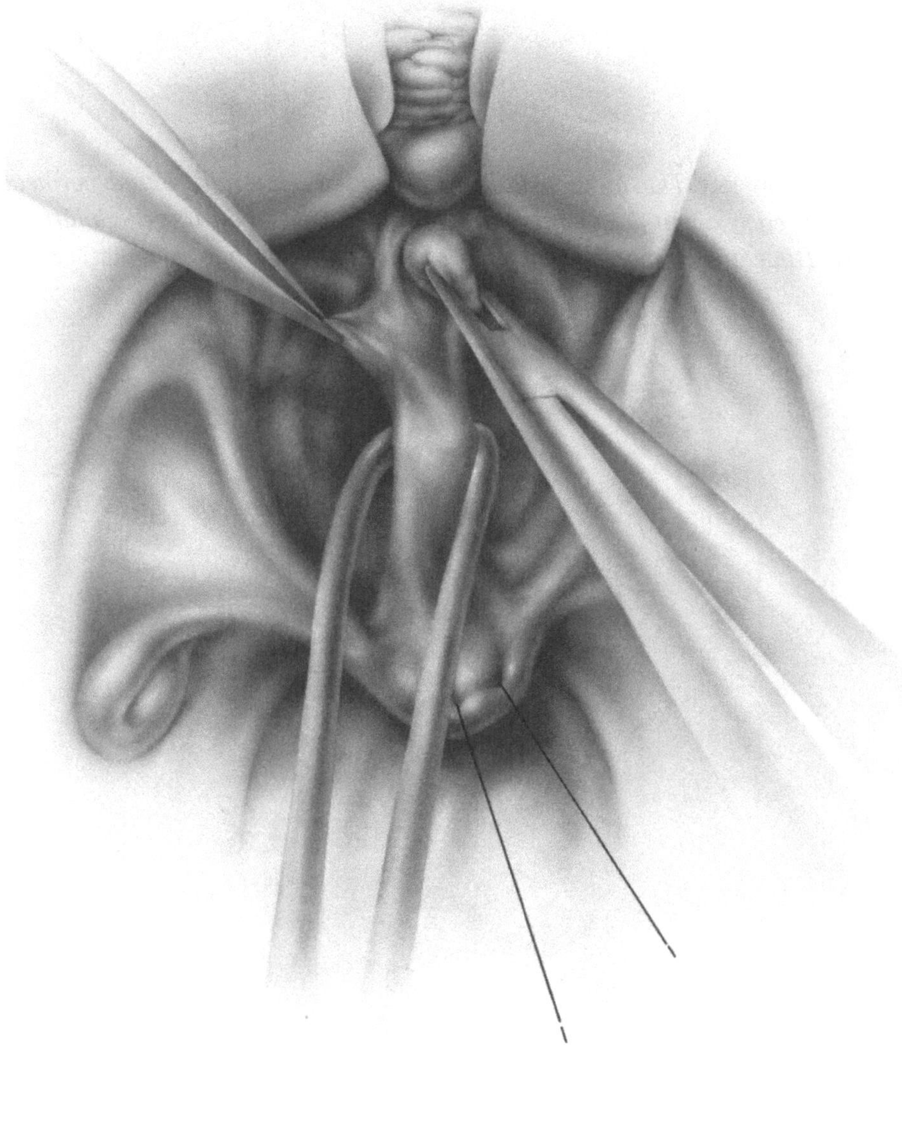

Fig. 12d. With tension on the sling, the anterior and posterior portions of the vagina are isolated by combined sharp and blunt dissection. The dissection is continued to the extent permitted by the laparotomy exposure. A head light must be used at this stage to illuminate the operative field. When the operator is unable to dissect further under vision, and abdominal towel is placed over the field, and attention is shifted to the perineum

Fig. 12e. Top left *The incision used to create two laterally based perineal skin flaps, each about 1–1.5 cm wide (or slightly wider in larger children).* Bottom *Dissection is carried out in a cranial direction between the urethra (UG sinus) and the rectum*

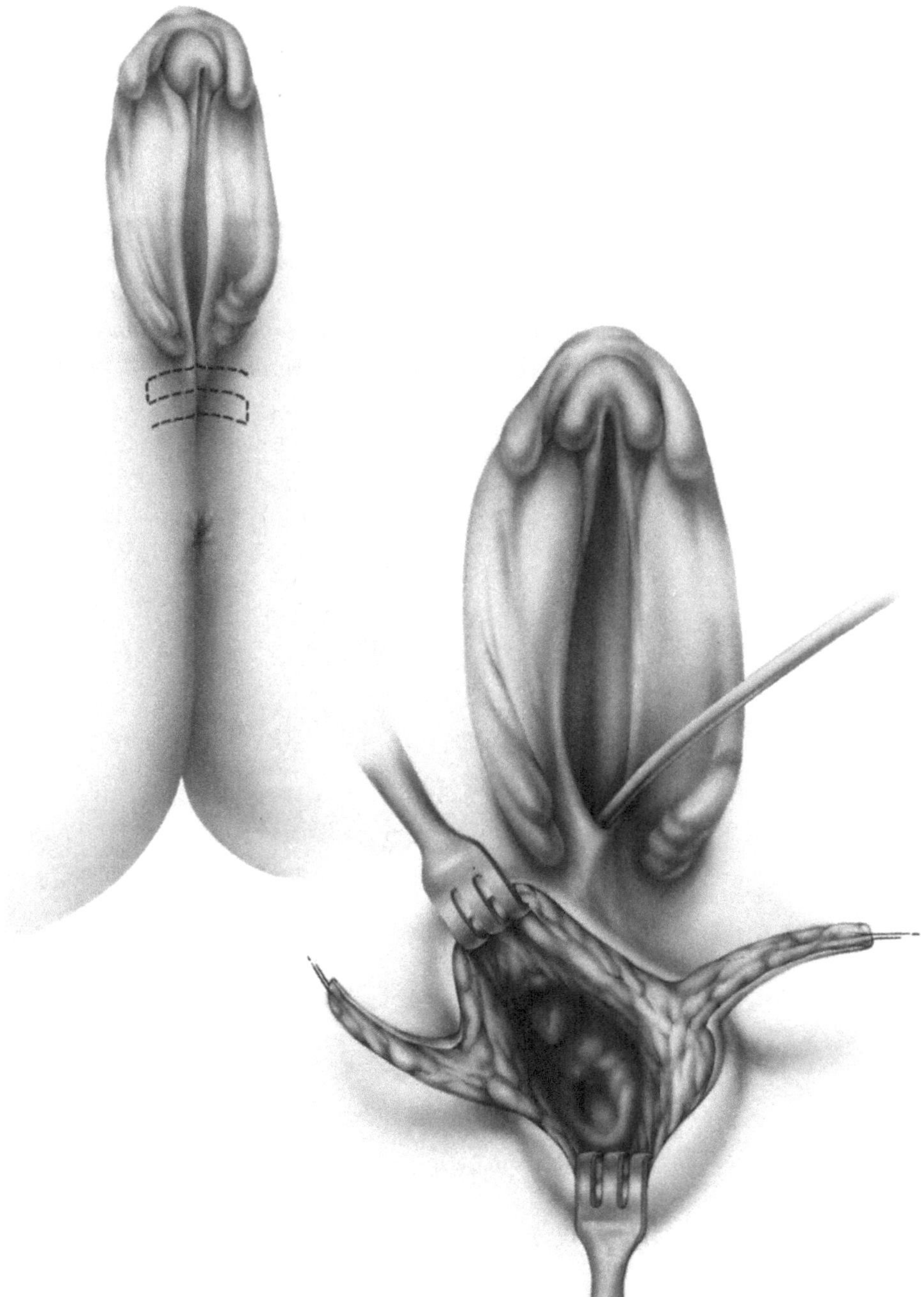

Fig. 12f. A dressing forceps is introduced into the abdomen from the perineal field, grasps the sling, and pulls it toward the perineum (left). *While this tension is maintained, the vagina is transected from the urogenital sinus in a stepwise fashion as stay sutures are placed through the vagina and the urethra (UG sinus) is closed* (bottom right). *All sutures are 6–0 Vicryl*

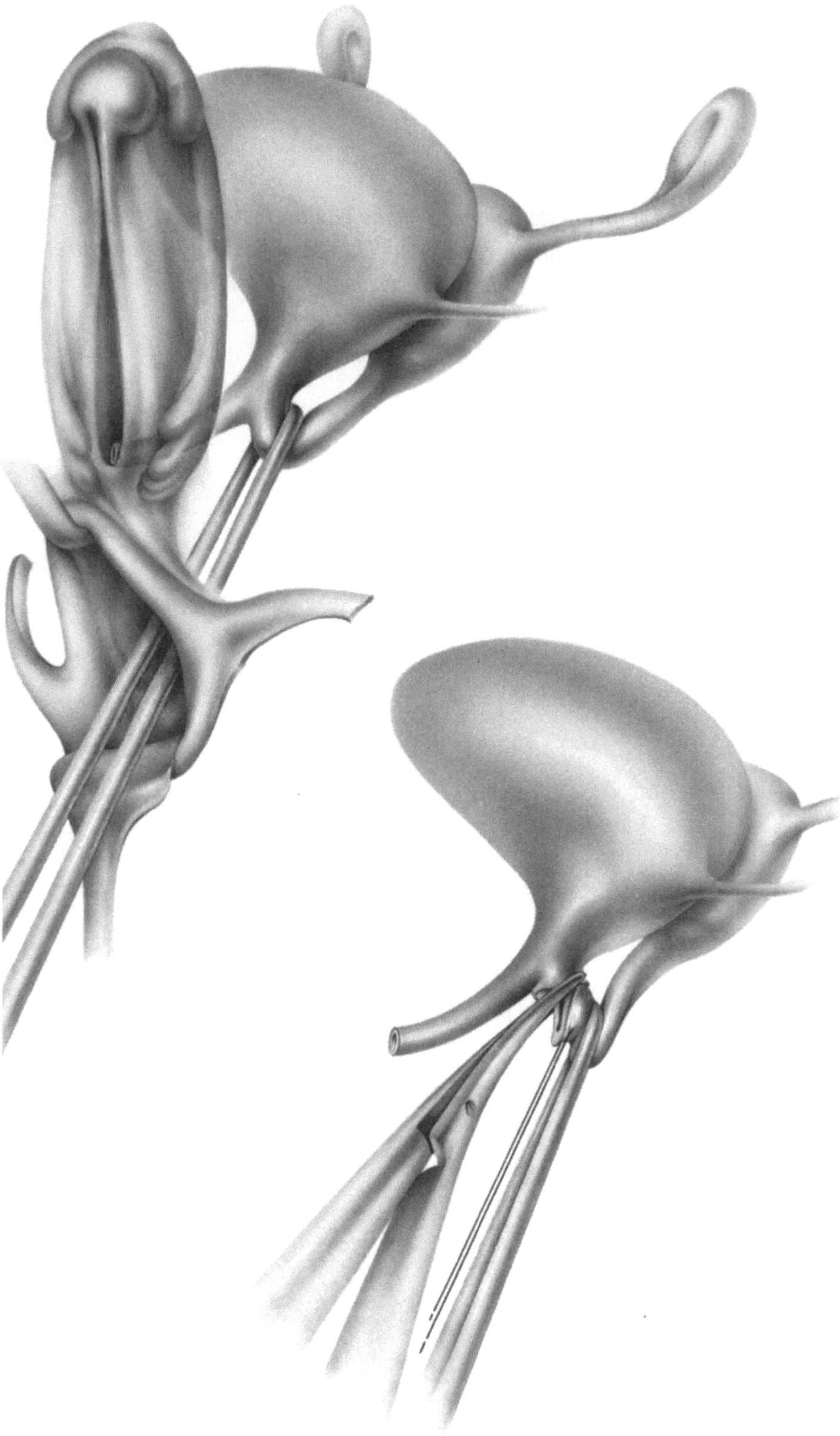

Fig. 12g. Status following detachment of the vagina from the urogenital sinus and closure of the urethral defect (left). *The detached vagina and urethral stump are visible in the perineal field* (right)

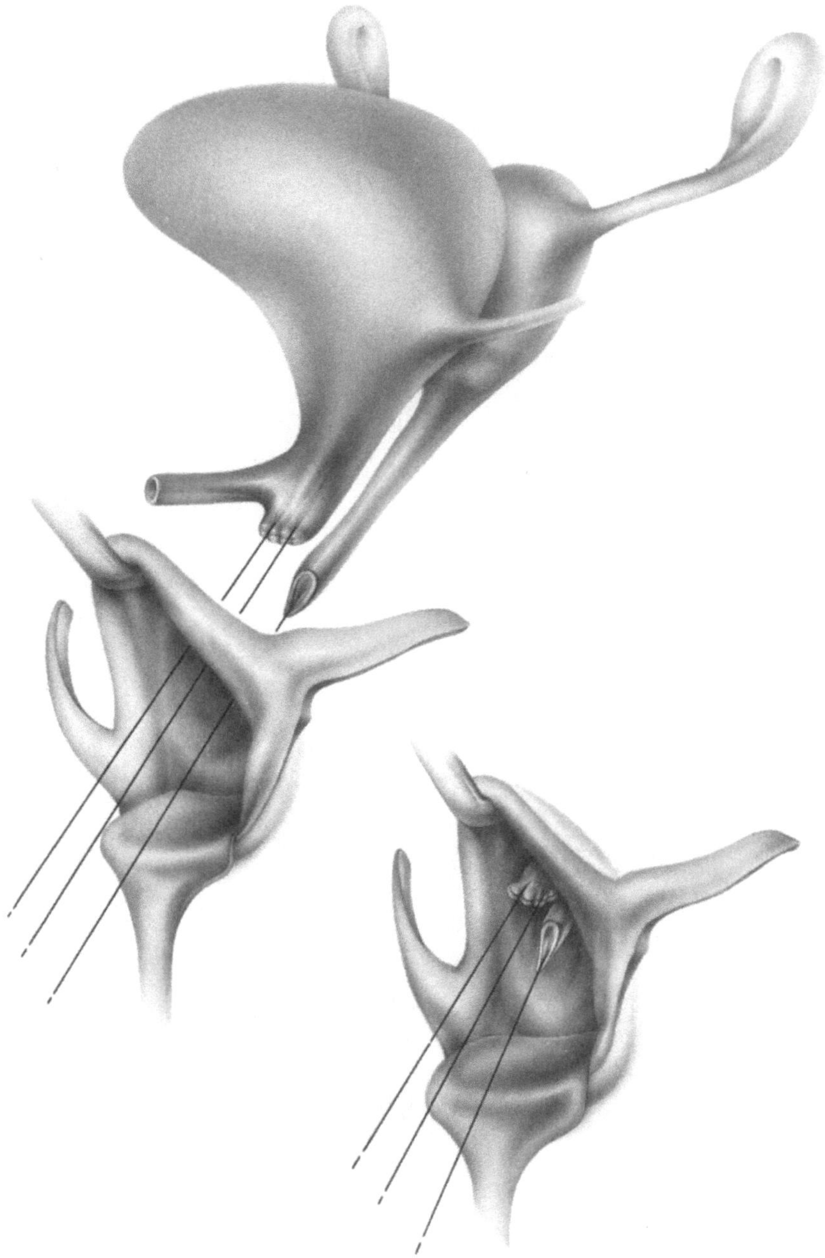

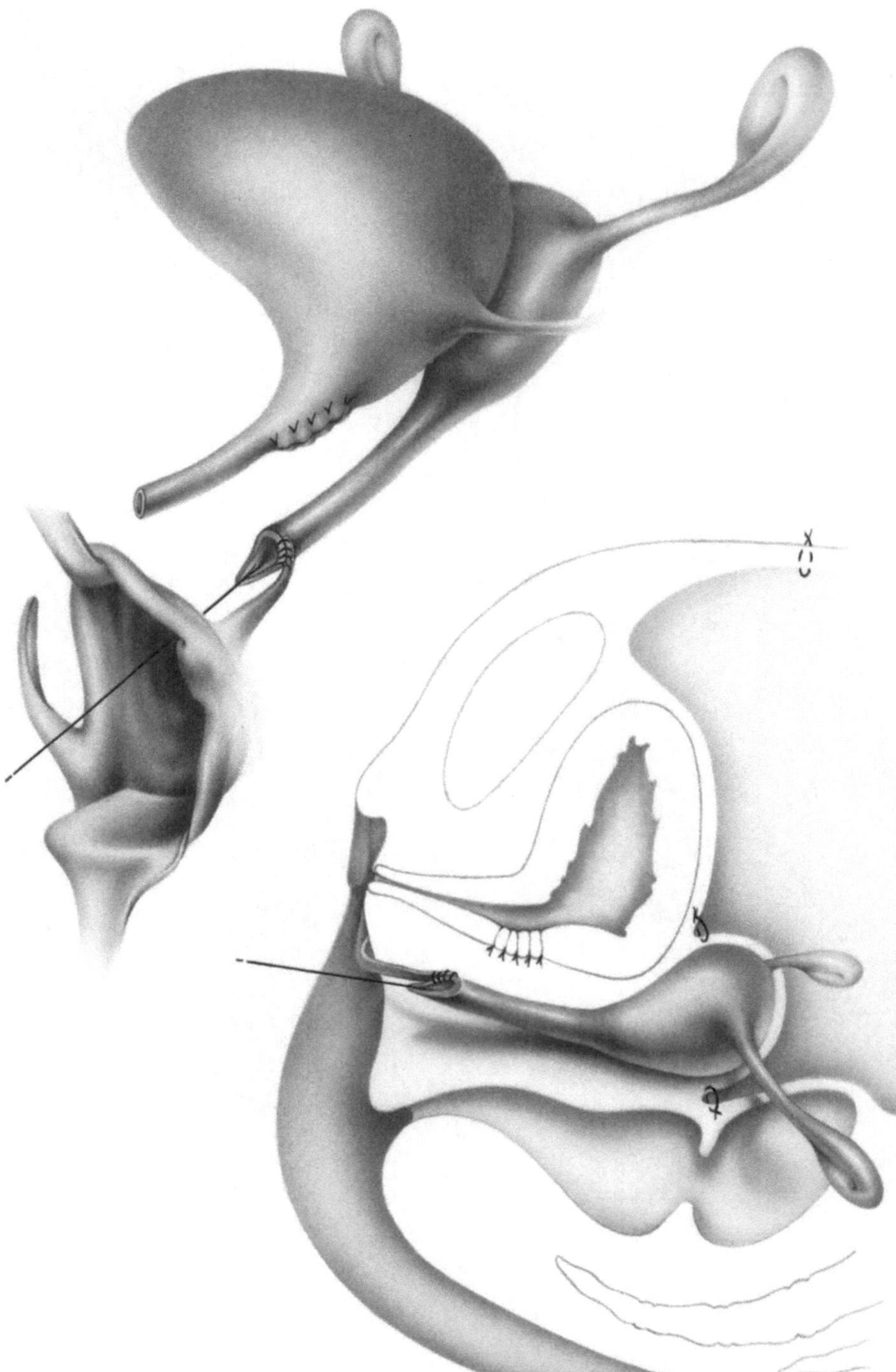

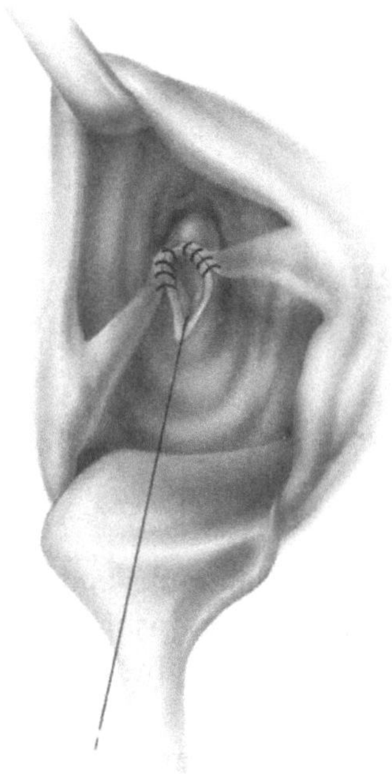

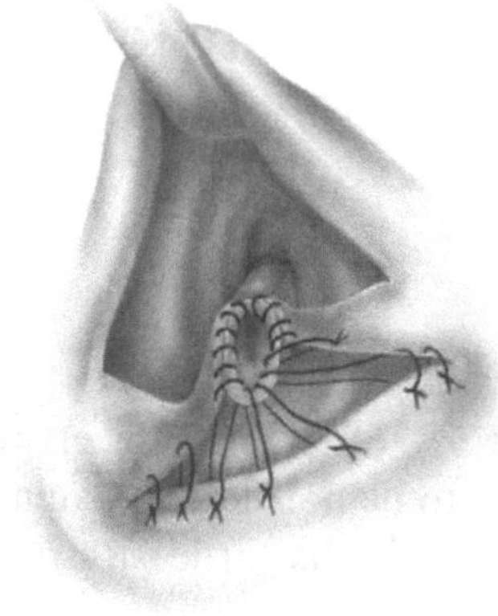

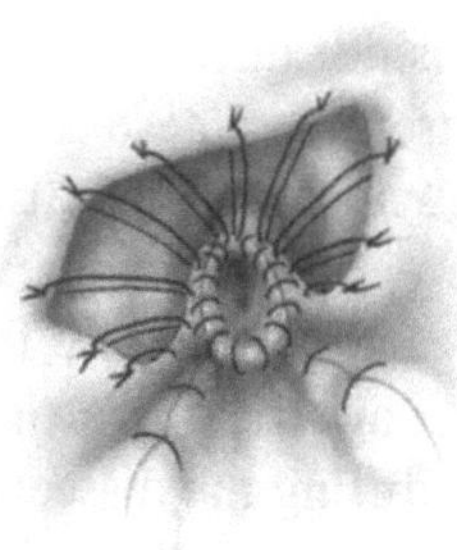

Fig. 12i. If the vagina is long enough, the skin flaps are apposed to the vagina about the full circumference of the vaginal orifice, which is additionally joined to the remaining wound edges of the perineal incision. If the vaginal tube is too short, the flaps are attached to the vaginal orifice with only 3 or 4 stitches, and the remaining wound edges are left open, as in Fig. 13b, c

←

Fig. 12h. The perineal skin flaps mobilized previously are anastomosed to the vagina with 7–0 Vicryl

Procedure for Subtotal Vaginal Aplasia

In about 5% of female subjects with AGS, contrast radiographs and endoscopy fail to demonstrate a vagina. If a uterus is found on ultrasonography, it is very likely that at least a rudimentary vagina is present. In these cases we proceed as follows:

The abdomen is opened with a Pfannenstiel incision, and the uterus is identified and engaged with a stay suture. The peritoneum is opened in the vesicouterine pouch and pouch of Douglas, and the vagina is dissected free. Given the extreme thinness of the vaginal wall, the dissection must proceed with meticulous care. It is not difficult to mobilize the vagina down to the region of the posterior urethra, where it terminates in a blind sac adherent to the urethra. The vagina is detached at that location. The operation is then continued from the perineum, where two laterally based skin flaps are created. Dissection is carried cranially from that point. A finger in the rectum and a Foley catheter aid the operator in identifying the rectum and urethra and protecting them during the dissection. The abdominal team marks the deepest point of the abdominal field with a dissecting patty, which is easily felt from the perineal side. After communication has been established between the abdominal and perineal fields, the abdominal team places two stay sutures through the uterus (Fig. 13), but not through the vagina, whose wall is usually too thin to retain a holding stitch. Once the sutures have been placed, the perineal team introduces a dressing forceps into the abdomen, grasps the stay sutures, and pulls the uterus and vagina down into the perineal field. At this time the previously mobilized perineal skin flaps are apposed to the vaginal inlet and sutured with 7-0 Vicryl. Due to the extreme thinness of the vaginal wall and the difficulty of placing sutures accurately deep within the perineal field, in two patients we have successfully joined the perineal flaps and vagina using only one suture per flap. In each case a vaginal stent is inserted to keep the vaginal channel distended after the flaps have been sutured. Even if only a narrow epithelial bridge is obtained between the vagina and perineum, complete epithelialization of the vaginal channel will ensue within a short time, similar to that occurring in the Denis Browne urethroplasty. To date we have had good results with this technique in six out of seven patients, with a satisfactory rate of vaginal growth. In one case the distal vagina became obliterated because the patient's parents had removed the stent prematurely.

The patients whom we have treated for partial vaginal aplasia were between 15 and 36 months of age, except for one child who was 8 years old at the time of surgery. Satisfactory growth of the vaginal canal was observed in seven children.

The gynecologic techniques of vaginal reconstruction described by McIndoe and Banister (1938), Wharton (1938), Counseller (1948), and Cali and Pratt (1968) are apparently designed only for patients with total vaginal aplasia, whereas our patients had only partial aplasias which allowed a connection to be established between the vestigial vagina and a perineal flap. The prevailing view of gynecologists that vaginoplasty should be postponed until regular coitus is desired is not appropriate for our surgical patients. A review of the older literature on vaginoplasties will reveal a study by the surgeon Kirschner and the gynecologist Wagner (1930), who created a neovagina by sewing a large Thiersch flap over a sponge prosthesis and inserting it into a tunnelized area between the rectum and urethra. Kirschner states that when the wound bed is completely covered by skin and the wound edges are accurately apposed, postoperative stenosis of the neovagina is not a problem, and he proves this in his study.

All our patients with partial vaginal aplasia had a urethra (urogenital sinus) which opened near the glans, corresponding to a Prader type IV anatomy. This necessitated a meatotomy, because the urinary stream on voiding was directed cranially rather than caudally following the clitoroplasty. We performed the meatotomy by introducing a fine, grooved probe into the distal urethra, incising the meatus for a length of 1 cm with a snip of the scissors, and suturing the epithelial border of the urethra to the skin (Vicryl). This enabled the patients to urinate well in the normal sitting position.

*Fig. 13a. The vagina and uterus in partial vaginal aplasia are mobilized through an abdominal approach as in Fig. 12a, b. A dressing forceps introduced into the abdomen from the perineal region is used to grasp the stay sutures in the body of the uterus (*not *the vagina) and pull it through to the perineum, delivering the vaginal opening into the perineal field*

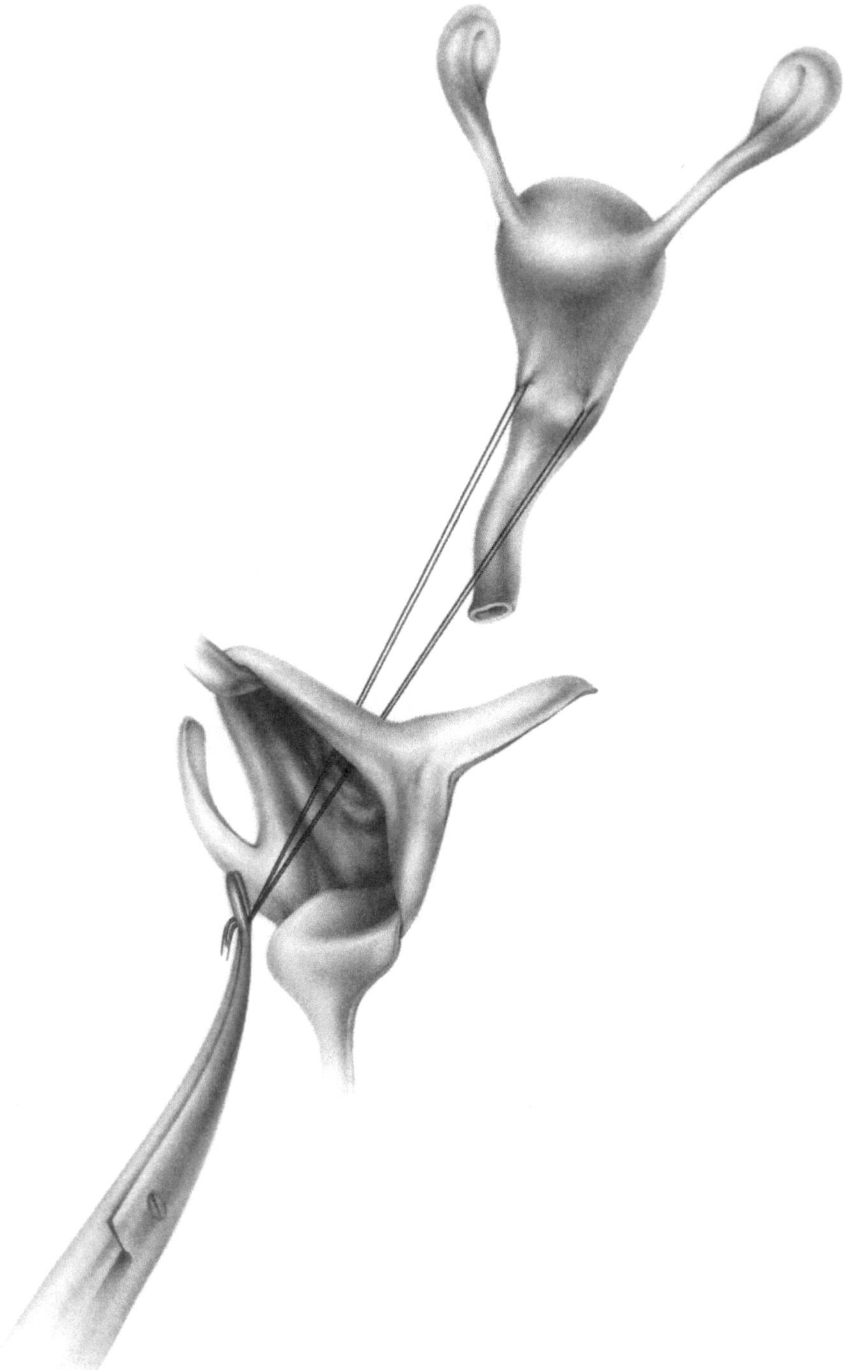

Fig. 13b. The perineal skin flaps are joined to the vagina, and a vaginal stent is inserted

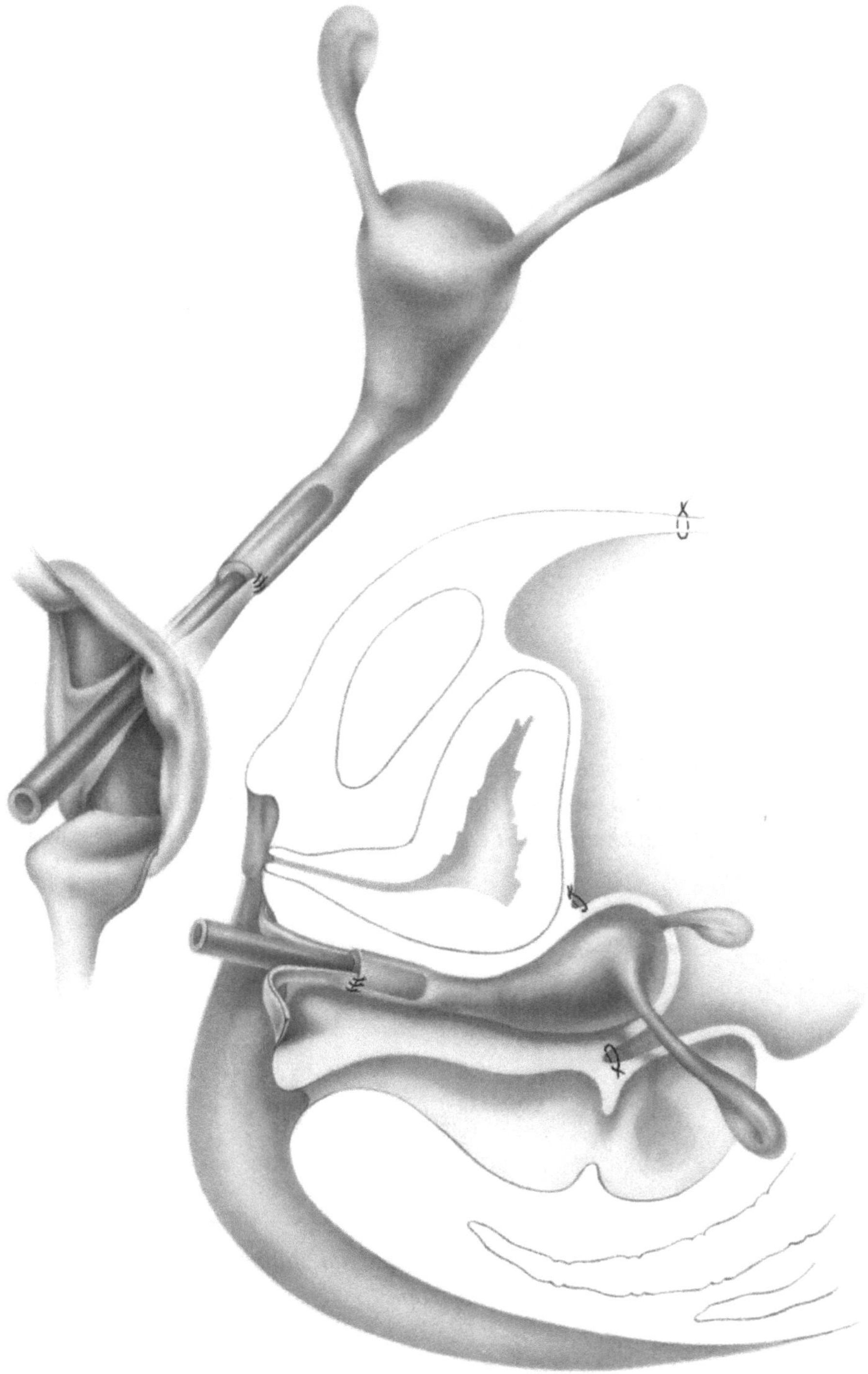

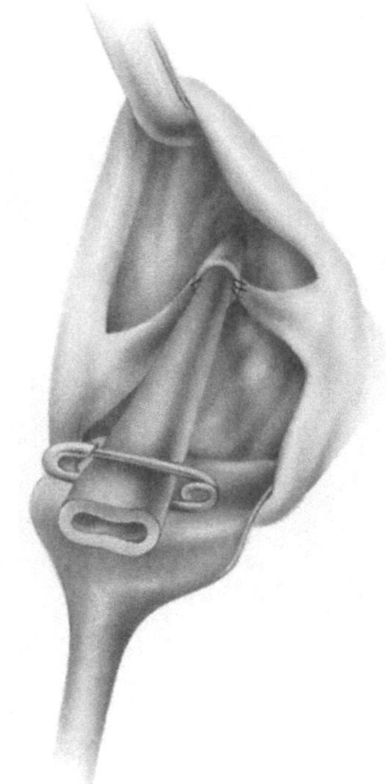

Fig. 13c. The operative field as viewed from the perineum, corresponding to Fig. 13b. If the vagina is too short, the remaining wound edges are left unsutured, and the soft-tissue channel will epithelialize completely within a few weeks

→

Fig. 13d. 18-Month-old AGS patient with partial vaginal aplasia and clitoral hypertrophy

Fig. 13e. A probe has been inserted to mark the urethral (UG sinus) opening. The external genitalia are Prader type IV

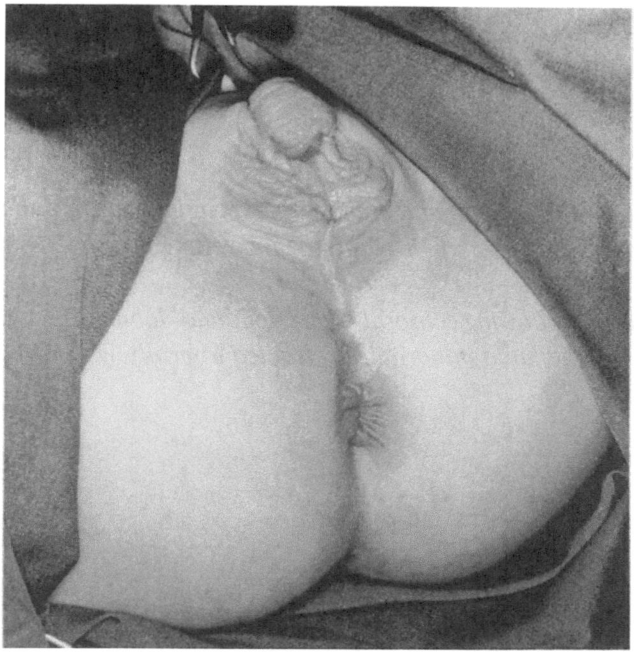

d

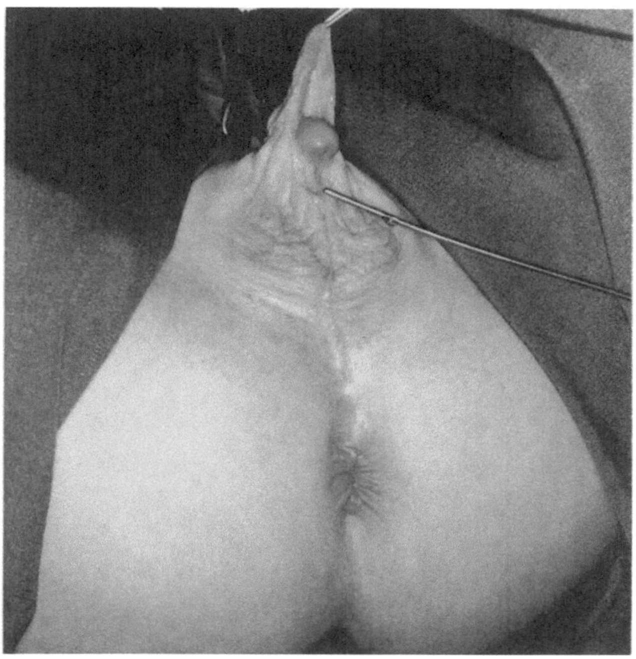

e

Fig. 13f. Status following an abdominoperineal vaginal pullthrough as described in Figs. 12 and 13. Note the indwelling vaginal stent

Fig. 13g. Status following clitoral recession and labioplasty according to Fig. 9. The labia minora are retracted laterally with forceps

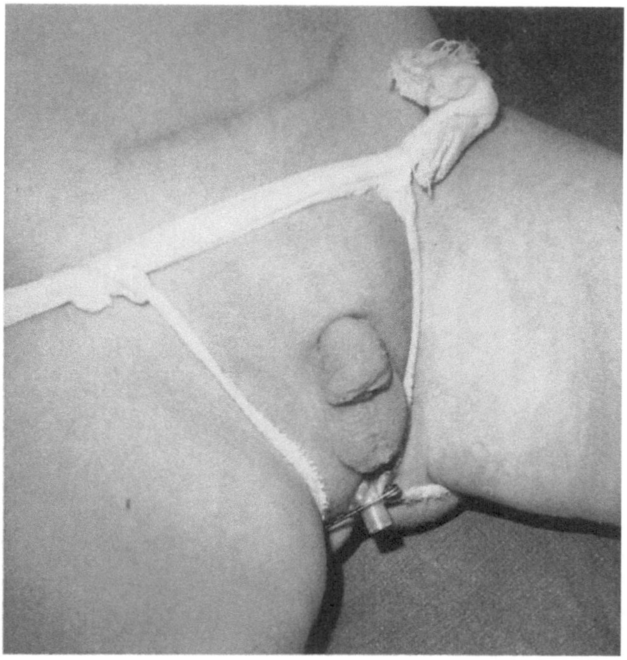

f

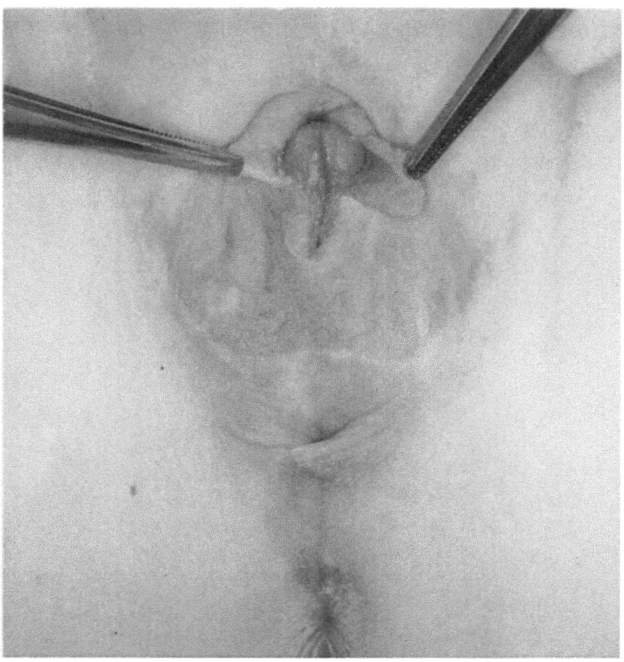

g

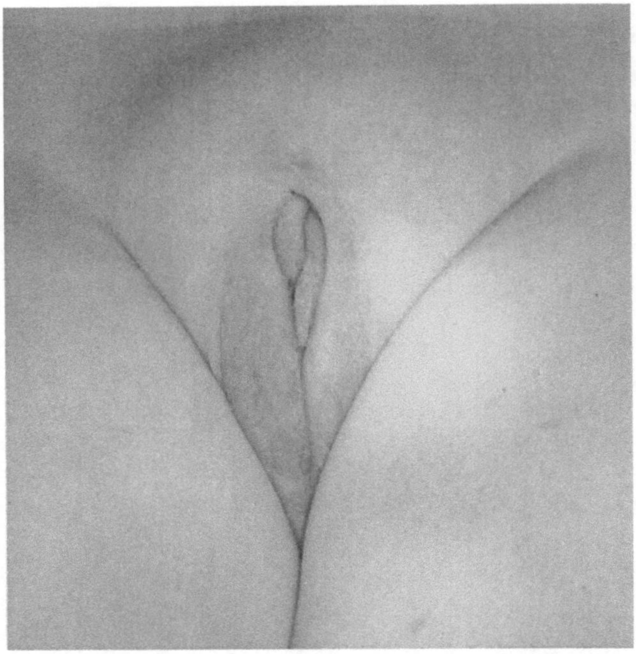

Fig. 13h. Appearance of the external genitalia with the legs adducted, demonstrating good coverage of the glans by the labia minora

Correction of Hydrometrocolpos Secondary to Hymenal or Vaginal Atresia

It should be possible to recognize hymenal atresia during the routine inspection of any newborn infant. Unfortunately, many of these children go undiagnosed until they present several years later, or even in early puberty, with an "abdominal mass" and intermittent abdominal pains. At this time a bulging, imperforate hymen is found on inspection of the genitalia. Excision of the hymen with closure of the wound margins (6-0 or 7-0 Vicryl) is the method of choice (Fig. 14). With a vaginal atresia, the diagnosis can be established and the level of the atresia identified by probing the vagina with a sound, combined if necessary with ultrasonography. Occasionally the vaginal obstruction will be missed by a superficial examination, and the surgeon will later discover the hydrometrocolpos while exploring for a "pelvic mass." Our technique of surgical correction is as follows (Fig. 15).

If the distal part of the vagina is atretic for up to 1 cm, the distended uterus or intraabdominal portion of the vagina is opened through a laparotomy, a small dressing forceps is advanced toward the perineum, and the lowest atretic part of the vagina is opened. The forceps is then advanced through the perineal incision and used to grasp a stent and pull it cranially until its proximal end rests in the upper vagina or uterus.

If the perineum and the atretic vagina are very far apart, two perineal skin flaps are created as shown in Fig. 12 and sutured to the vagina.

We have found that the wound bed epithelializes completely within a few weeks after this surgery, and that the formerly atretic part of the vagina does not contract, but grows satisfactorily (Fig. 16).

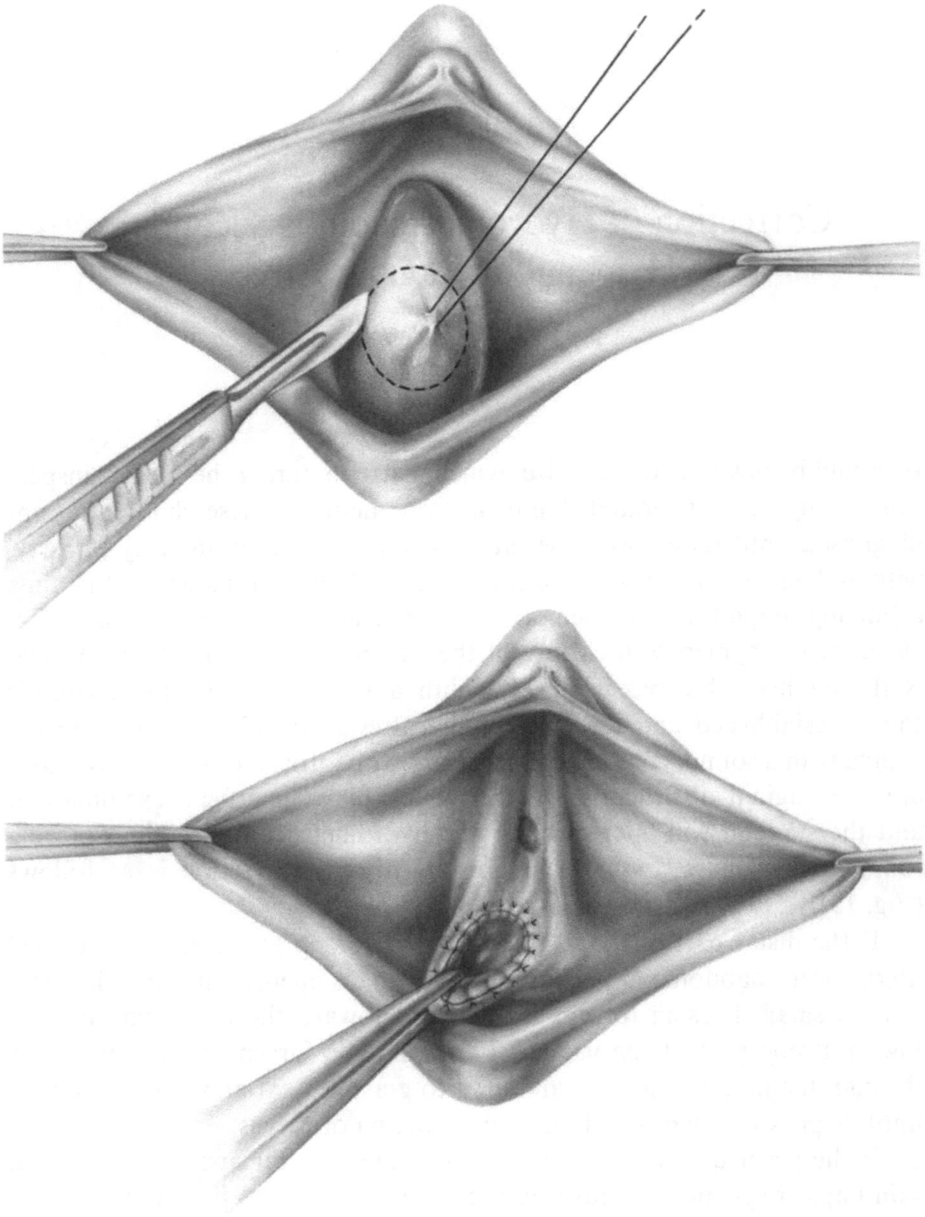

Fig. 14a. To correct complete hymenal atresia, a stay suture is placed at the center of the hymen, a circular hymenal segment is excised, and the vaginal epithelium is joined to the vulvar epithelium with vertical mattress sutures of 7–0 Vicryl. The vagina is tamponaded with a tulle strip for 3 days

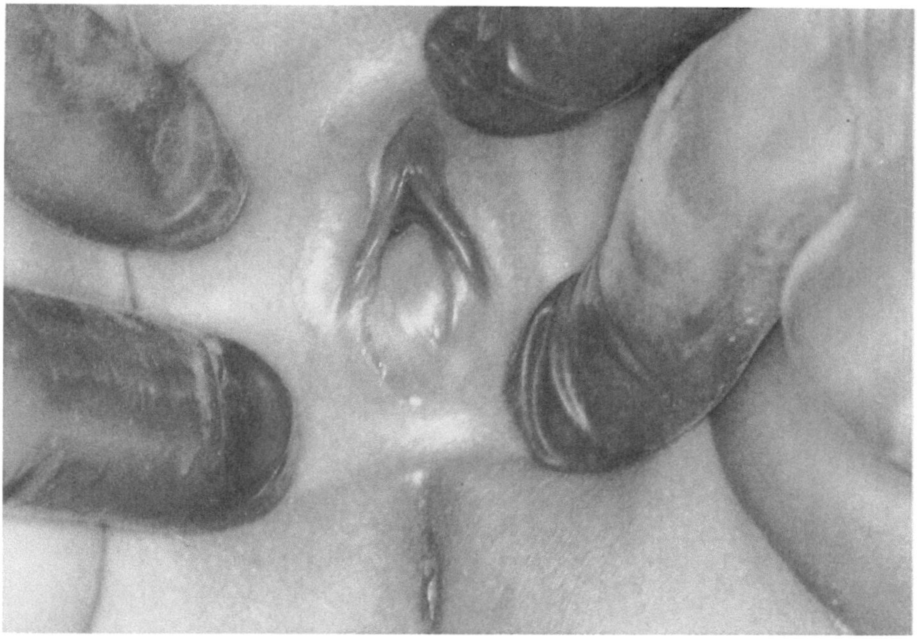

Fig. 14b. One-month-old girl with hymenal atresia and hydrometrocolpos

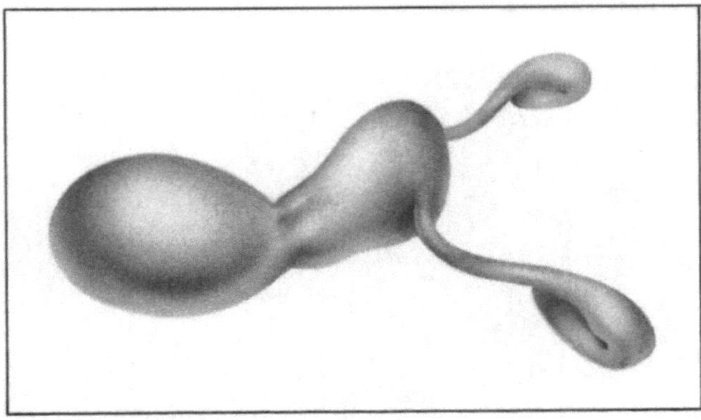

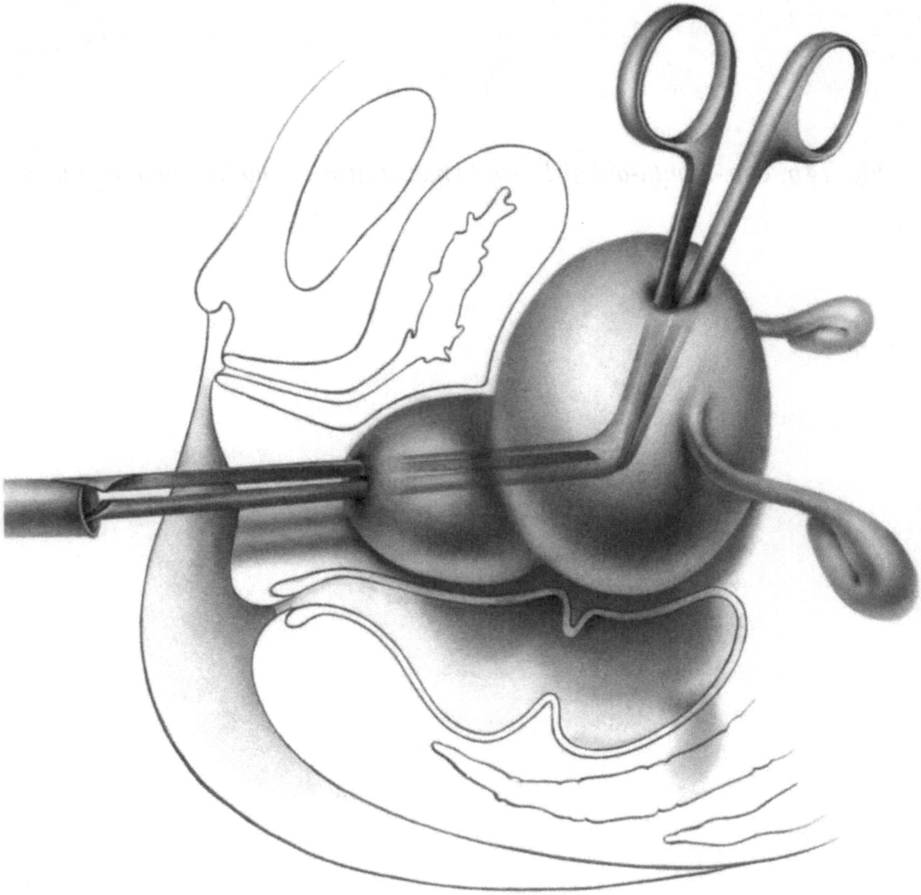

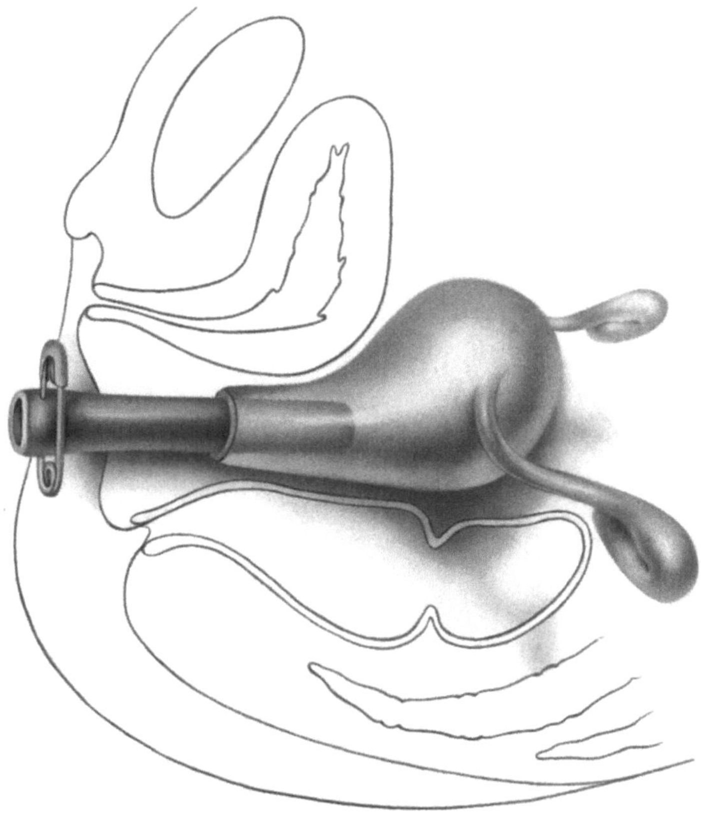

Fig. 15b. The vaginal stent in situ. A tube of vaginal epithelium will form along the stent within a few weeks, creating a neovagina that will grow with the patient, as numerous observations have proved

←

Fig. 15a. To correct hydrometrocopolpos, the widely distended uterus is opened through a laparotomy incision, and the uterine contents are aspirated. A perineal incision is made, and an angled dressing forceps is inserted into the uterus through the abdominal incision, perforating the vaginal sac at its lowest point and grasping a stent through the perineal incision. The stent is then drawn into the vagina

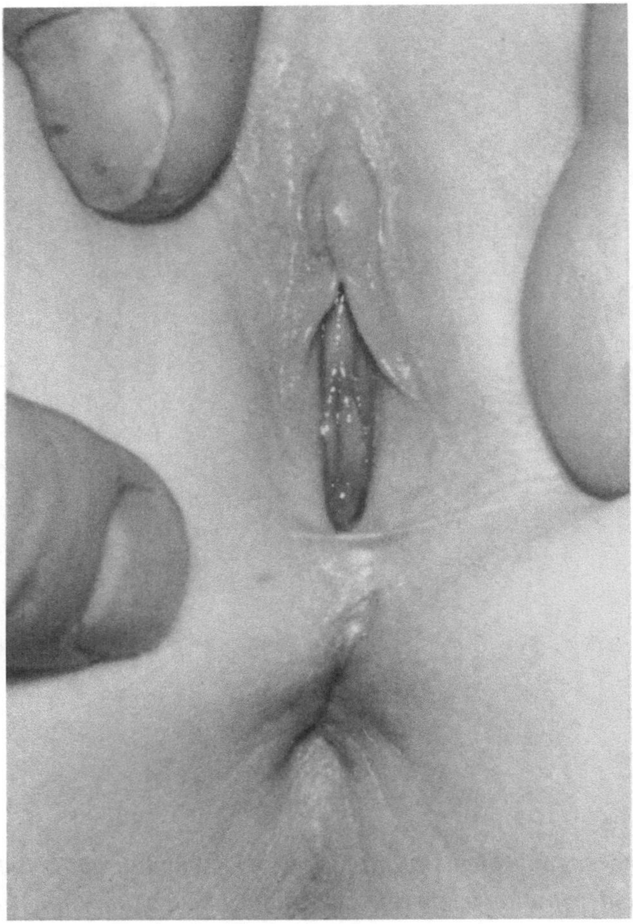

a

Fig. 16a, b. Six-year-old girl who underwent surgical correction for distal vaginal aplasia and hydrometrocolpos. (a) The vaginal introitus appears normal; (b) a No. 10 Hegar dilator is introduced without difficulty. The vagina shows a satisfactory rate of growth

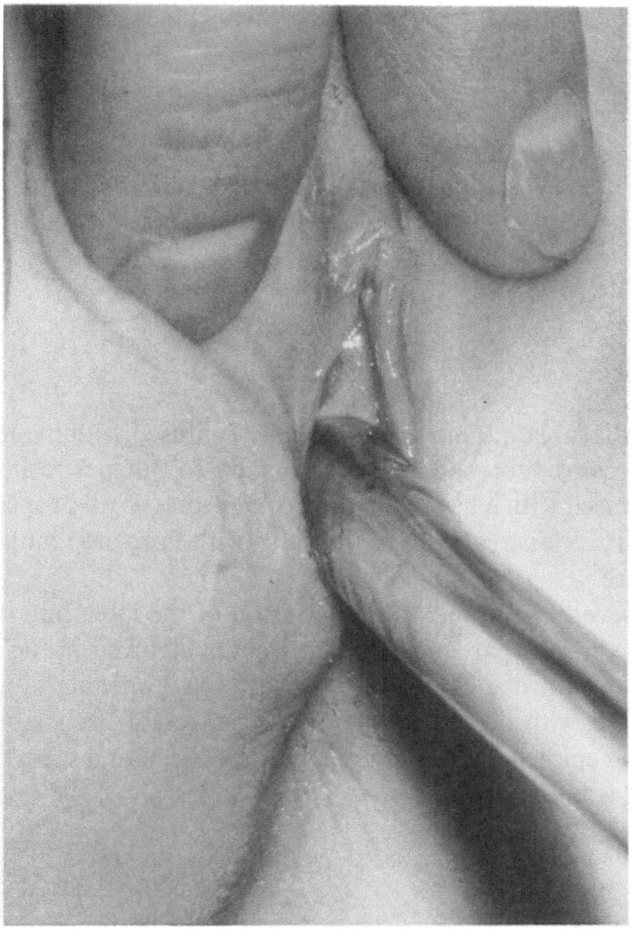

b

Synechia of the Labia Minora

Synechia of the labia minora is occasionally confused with hymenal atresia. Most cases involve labial adhesions secondary to "diaper rash," and most are easily released with a dissecting forceps or probe. With proper anogenital hygiene and 1 week's treatment of the vulva with Progynon ointment, recurrences are rare.

A more severe abnormality is true fusion of the labia minora (Fig. 17). However, the cranial part of the labia is never involved in the fusion, and so a fine grooved probe can be inserted into this "opening" and the fused labia separated with a scalpel. The incised edges of each labium (vulvar and cutaneous epithelium) are sutured with 7-0 Vicryl and sealed with bucrylate. Healing is uneventful.

Fig. 17. Fusion of the labia minora is corrected by introducing a grooved protector, incising the fused tissue over the protector, and closing the wound edges (vulvar epithelium and skin) with vertical mattress sutures of 7-0 Vicryl

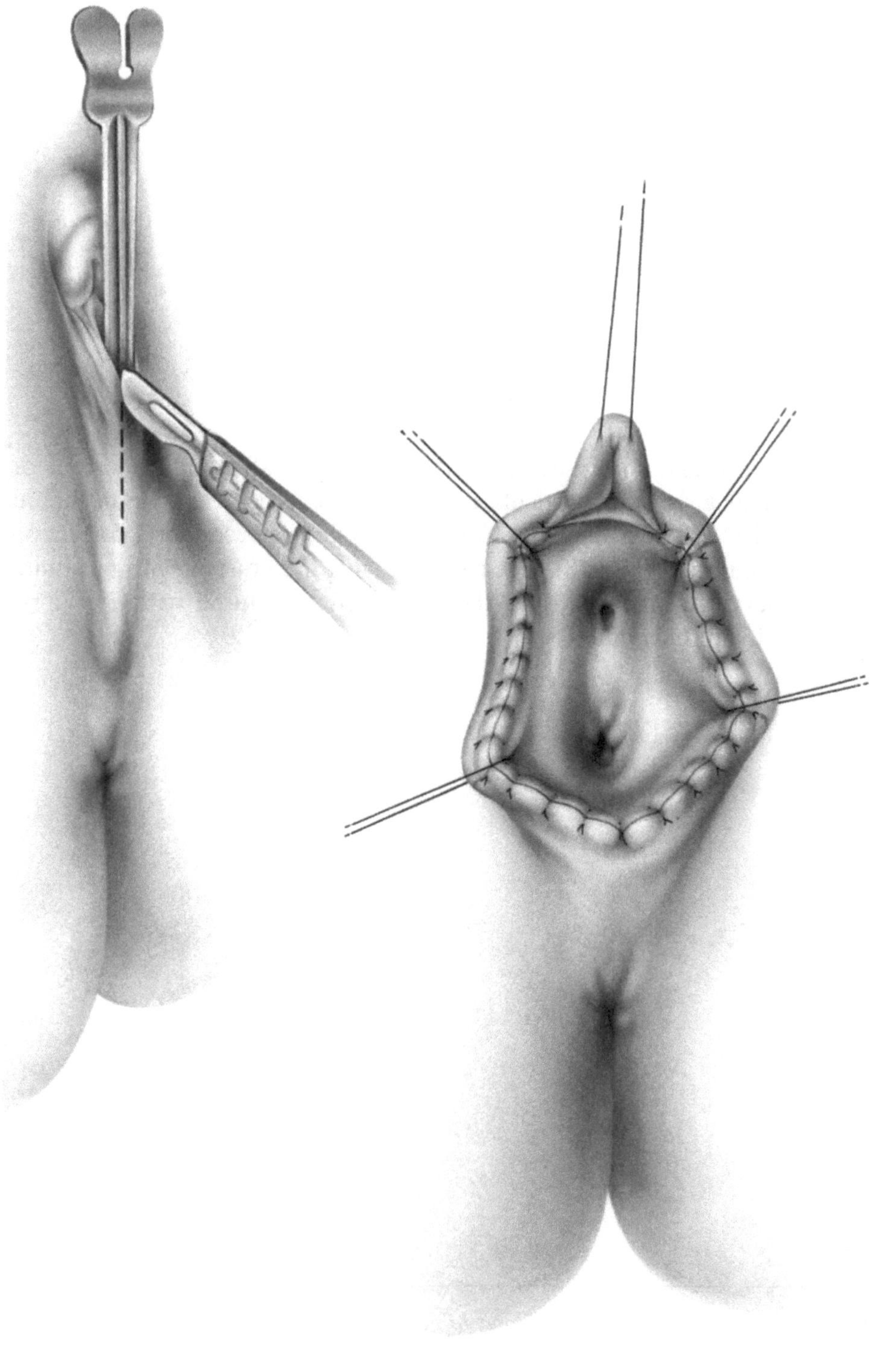

Hypertrophy of the Labia Minora

This is a rare and sometimes grotesque condition affecting pubescent or prepubescent girls. It is particularly common in Africa but also occurs at our latitudes. Whether the hypertrophy is primary or secondary, correction is always indicated (Fig. 18). The enlarged labia are grasped with mosquito clamps, surgically reduced, and the wound edges sutured with 7-0 Vicryl and sealed with bucrylate.

Fig. 18a. To correct hypertrophied labia minora (pudendal apron), the labia are engaged with clamps and stay sutures, excess tissue is resected, and the wound edges are approximated with 7–0 Vicryl following careful hemostasis;

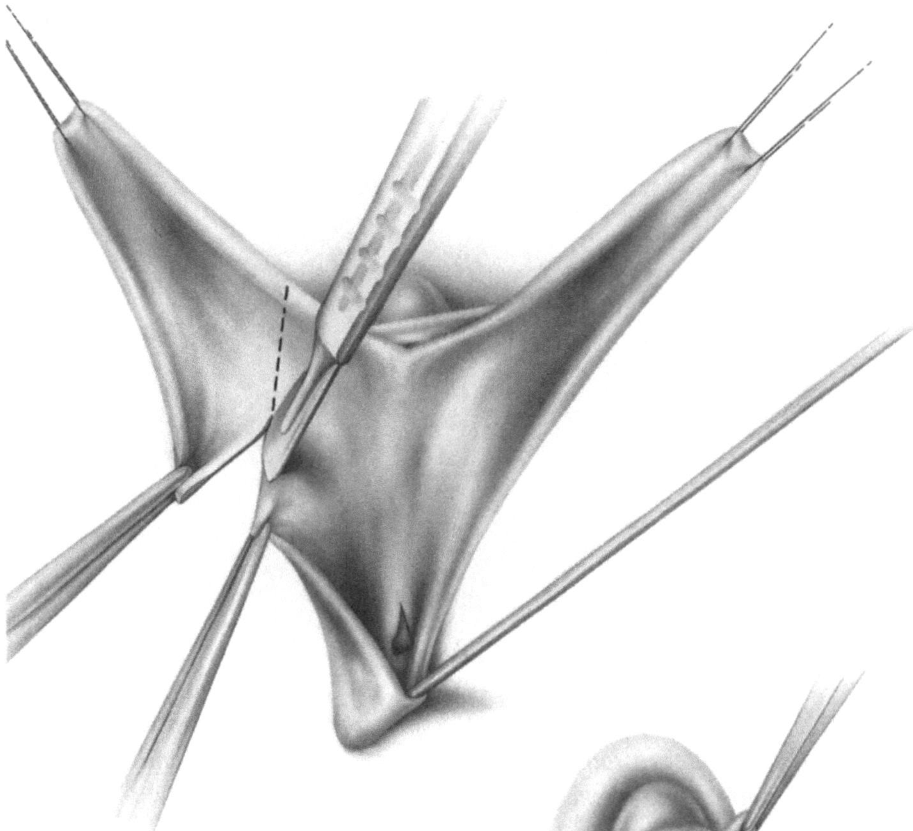

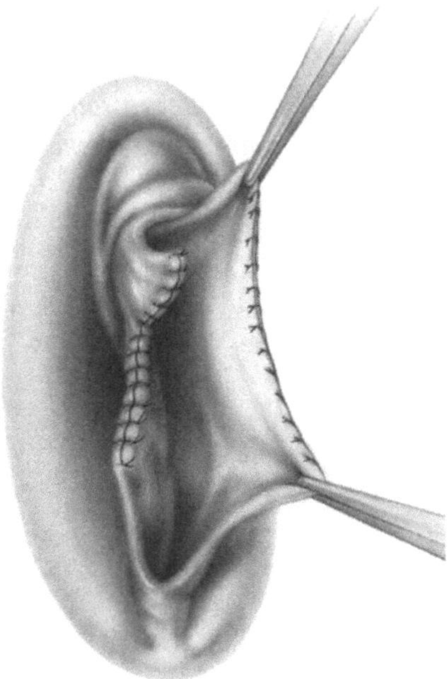

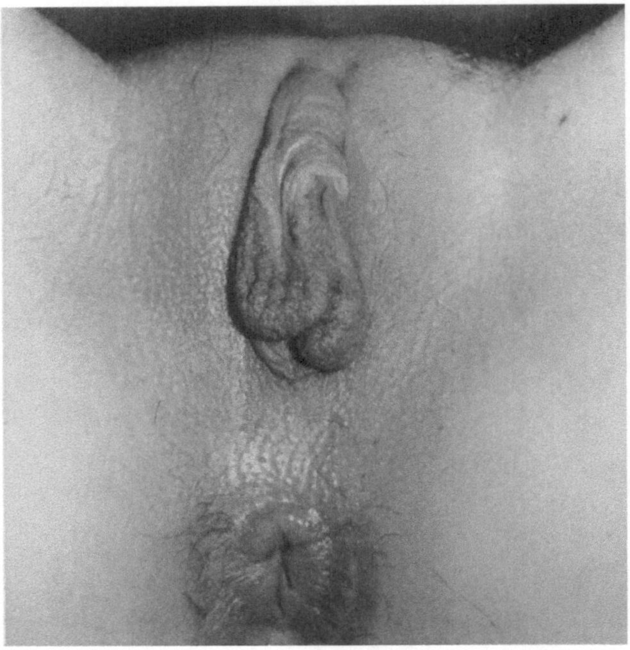

b

Abb. 18b–d. (b) 13-year-old girl with hypertrophied labia minora; (c) the hypertrophied labia are unfolded (patient is shaved in (a) and (b): (d) appearance of the genitalia 6 months postoperatively

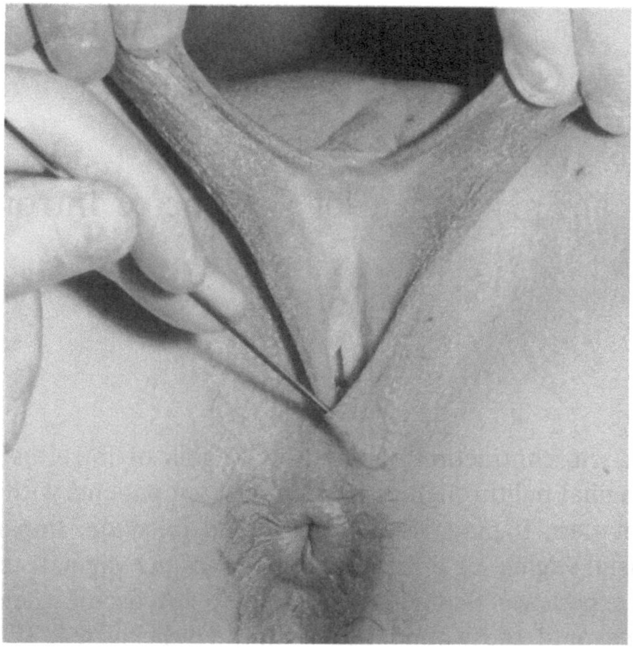

c

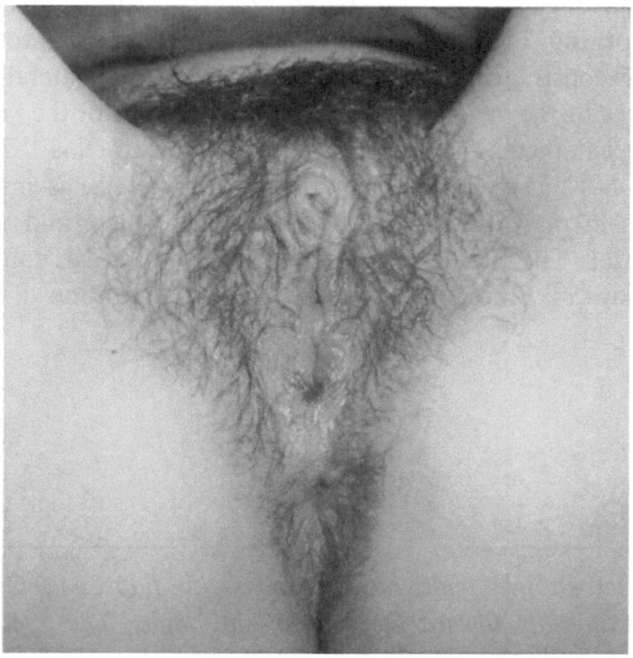

d

Surgical Enlargement of Contracted Introitus

While uncommon, contraction of the distal vagina or introitus is possible following a vaginal pullthrough or introitoplasty in patients with urogenital sinus malformation. It may result from wound infection, impaired blood flow to the distal vagina, or premature removal of the vaginal stent.

It is our experience that contraction does not occur when the stent is left in place until the wound bed is fully epithelialized. If a stricture does develop, we recommend the following technique of correction (Fig. 19):

A pair of elongated, caudally based skin flaps are created lateral to the vaginal opening. The cranial flap incisions are extended into the vagina such that the constricted part of the vagina is incised laterally on each side. The edges of the vaginal incision are separated until the vaginal tube is adequately enlarged. The skin flaps are swung into this "defect" and sutured with 6-0 Vicryl, and a stent of appropriate size is inserted. The stent remains in place until wound healing is complete and all surfaces are epithelialized. The flap donor sites are sutured with fine, nonabsorbable suture material (5-0 Ethibond) following slight mobilization of the wound edges.

Fig. 19a. We create two anally based perineal skin flaps, each 2–3 cm wide, which extend laterally toward the bend of the thighs. The exact length of the flaps depends on the degree of the vaginal stricture. The solid lines *at the vaginal introitus indicate that the incisions are carried into the vagina down to the end of the stricture*

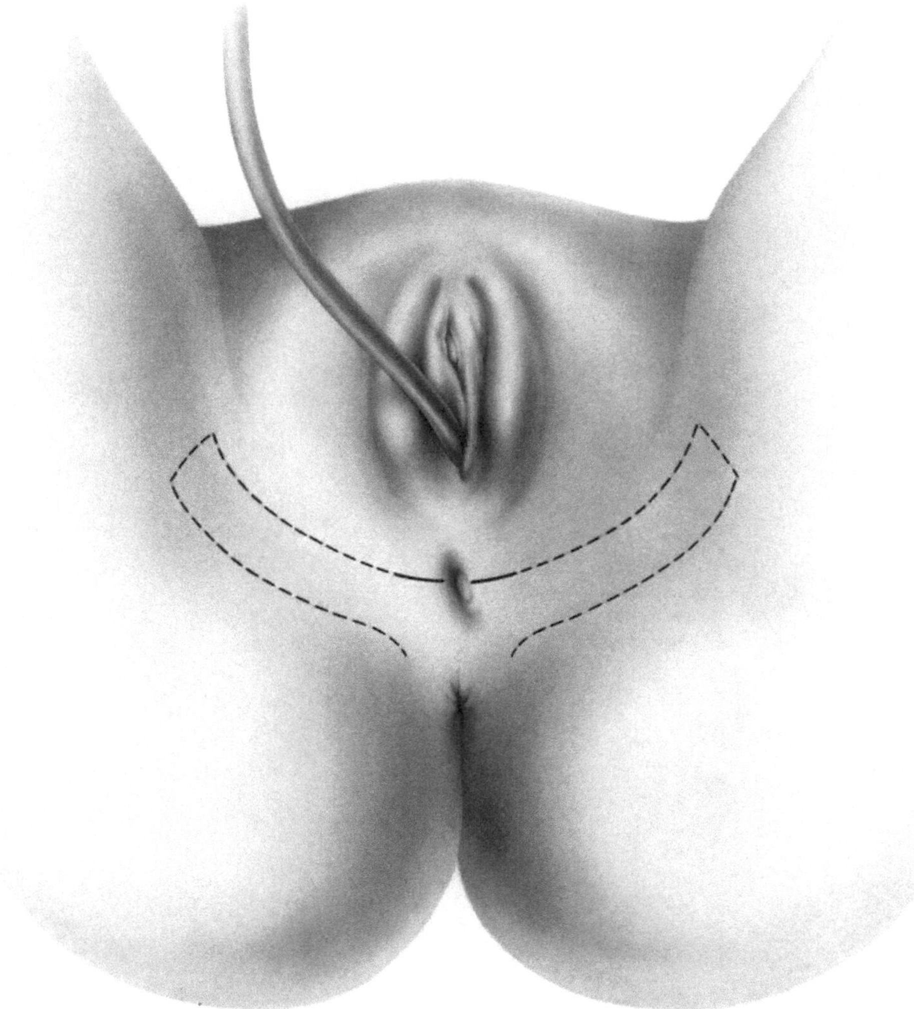

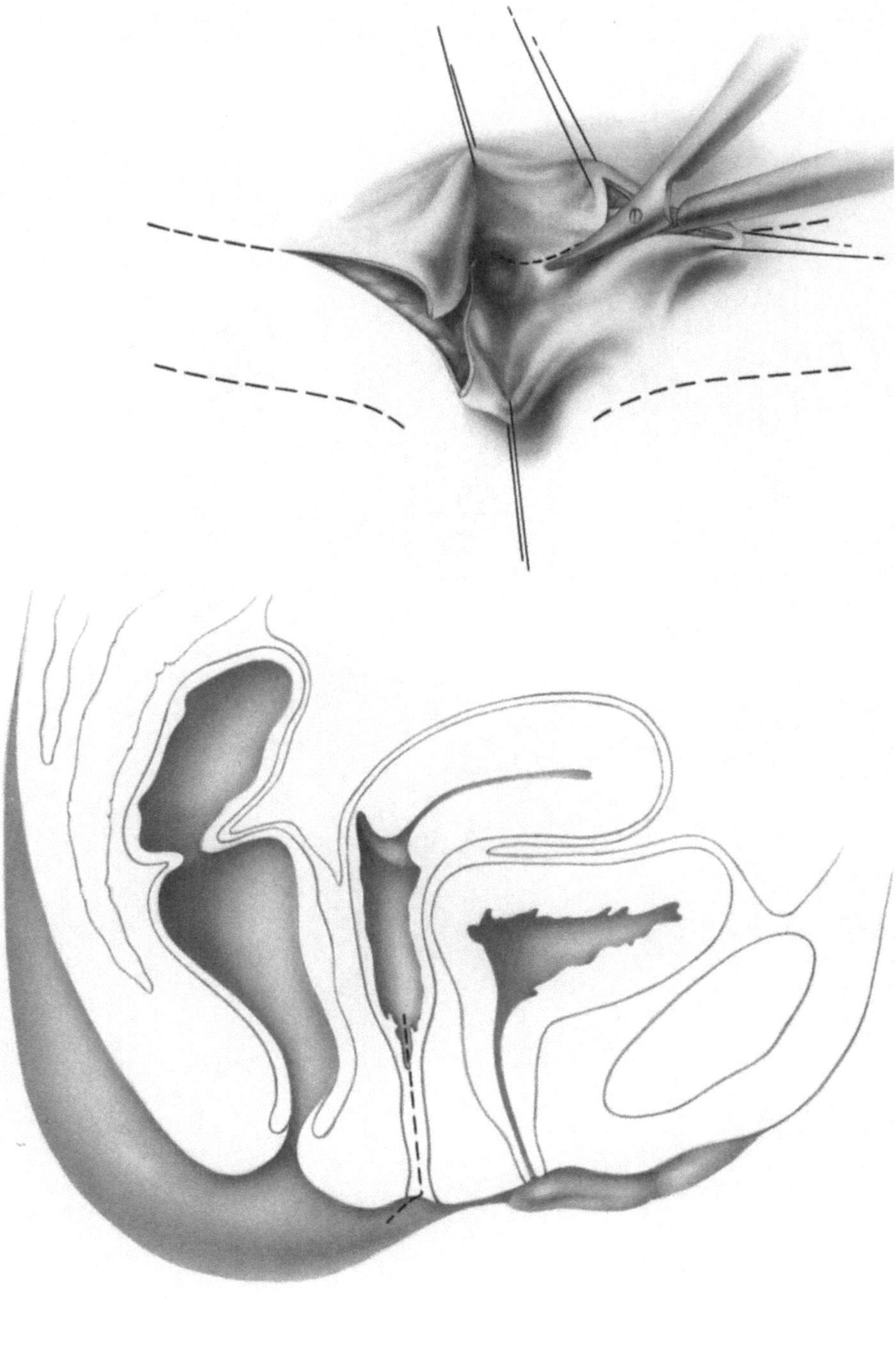

Fig. 19b. The lines of incision as seen from the AP (top) *and lateral views* (bottom)

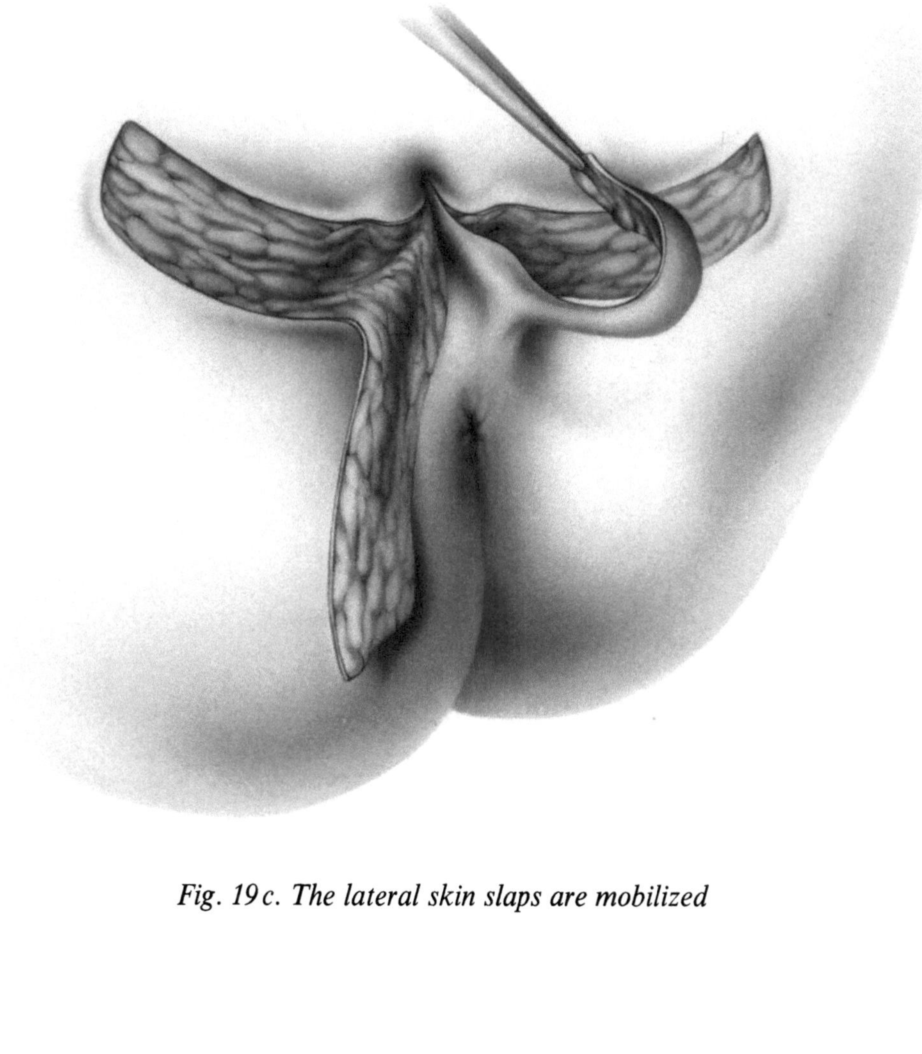

Fig. 19c. The lateral skin slaps are mobilized

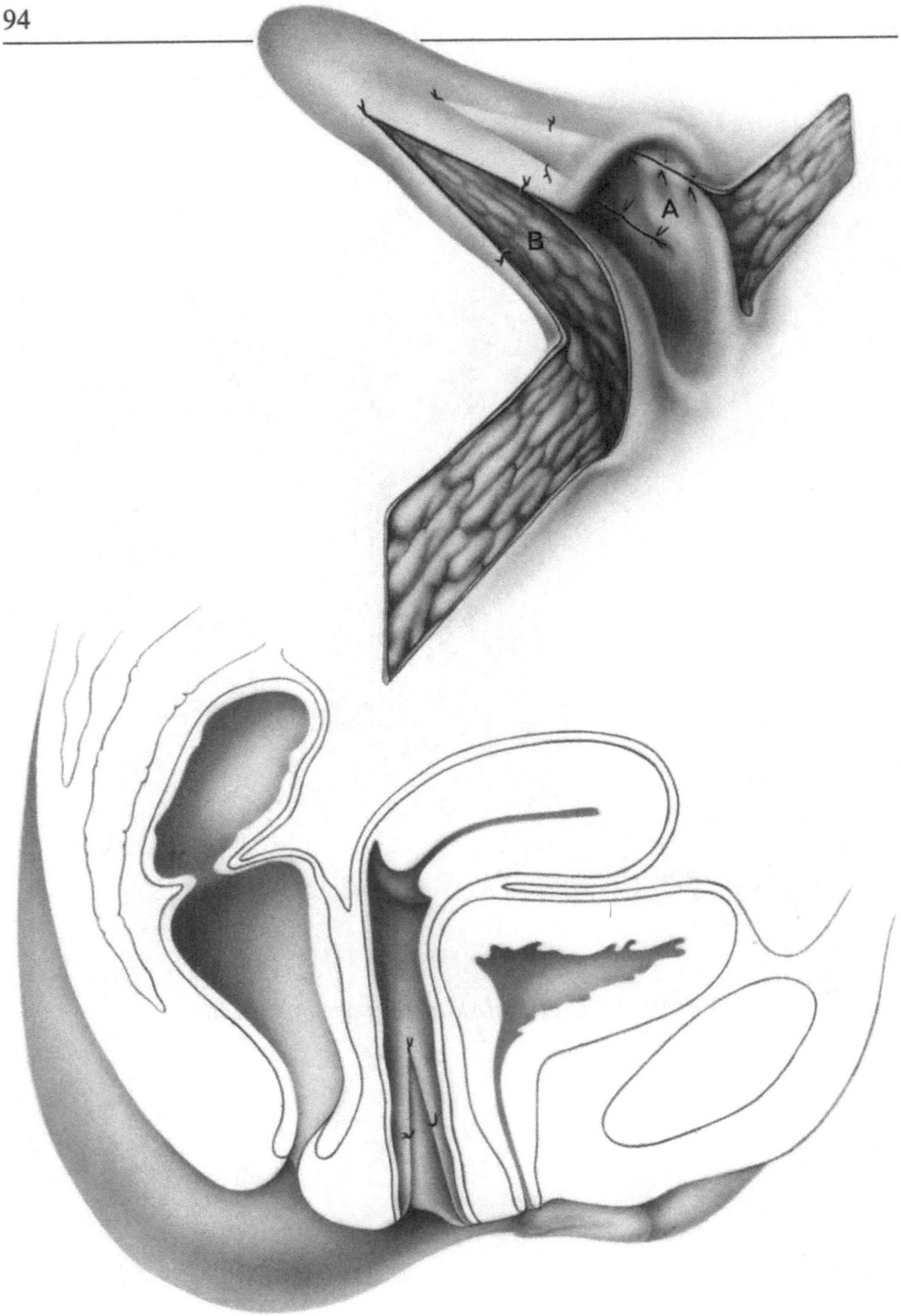

Fig. 19d. The mobilized skin flaps are advanced into the vagina and into the defect to enlarge the vaginal inlet (top) *and are sutured with 6–0 Vicryl.* Bottom *cross-sectional view of the vaginoplasty*

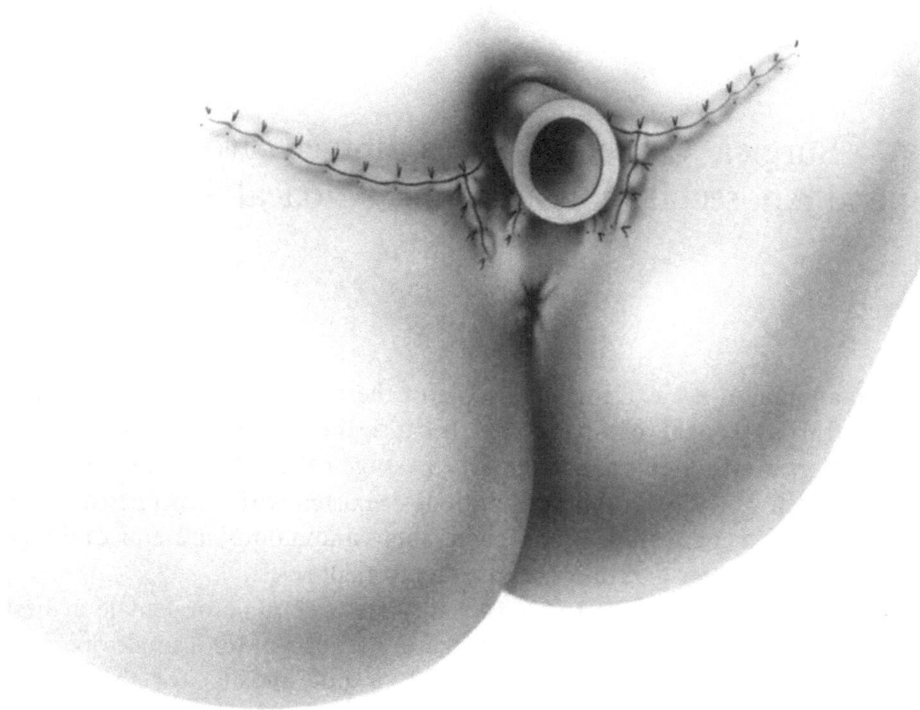

Fig. 19e. Postoperative appearance of the vaginoplasty with the stent in place

Surgical Correction of Combined Urogenital and Anorectal Malformations (Cloacal Syndrome)

These anomalies are extremely variable in their form. They are sometimes referred to as cloacal malformations, because the urethra, vagina, and rectum all open into a common excretory passage called the cloaca. We have seen cases in which cloacal malformations coexisted with hydrometrocolpos and extreme megarectum. Many cases show anomalous ureteral drainage with a megaloureter and in some cases hydronephrosis.

Often it is not possible to identify the infant as male or female at first evaluation, for the perineum is largely featureless except for a single opening, which may be at the tip of a phallus. It is not unusual for these cases to be misdiagnosed as anorectal atresia with hypospadias. Genetic evaluation is mandatory. In most cases the cloacal malformation can be diagnosed preoperatively on the basis of sonography and contrast films obtained with a catheter passed through the meatus (Fig. 20).

→

Fig. 20 a, b. Radiographic demonstration of a cloacal syndrome in the lateral projection. (a) A catheter is inserted into the bladder and another into the rectum. Left *As contrast medium is first injected, a broad space becomes visible between the urethral and rectal catheters. Already the air-filled vagina and cervical fossa can be appreciated.* Right *The rectum and bladder are well demonstrated. (b)* Left *The rectum, sigmoid colon, and urinary bladder are well filled. The catheter is withdrawn to fill the vaginal opening with contrast medium and visualize the cervix.* Right *The bladder is well filled, the urethra is delineated, and the vagina, rectum, and rectocloacal fistula are well demonstrated*

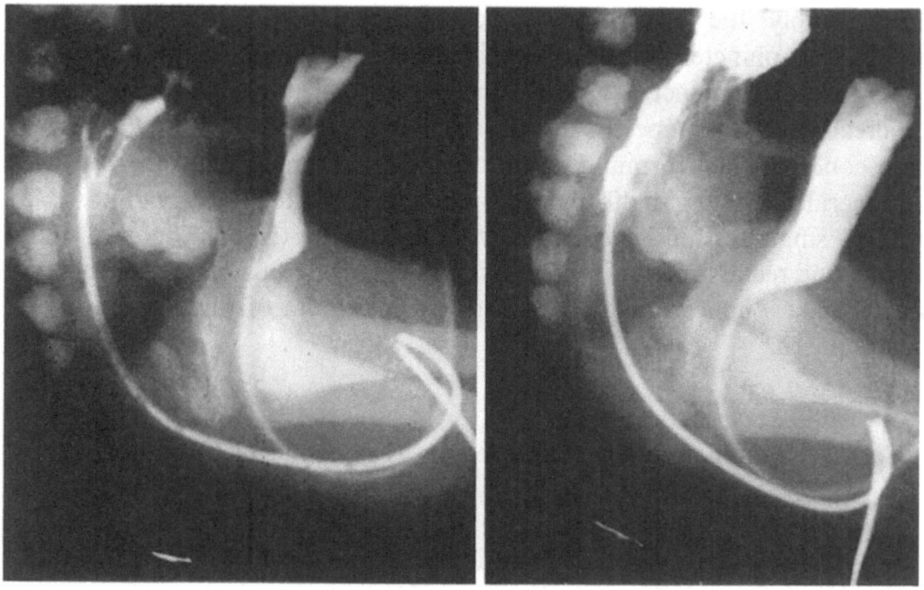

a

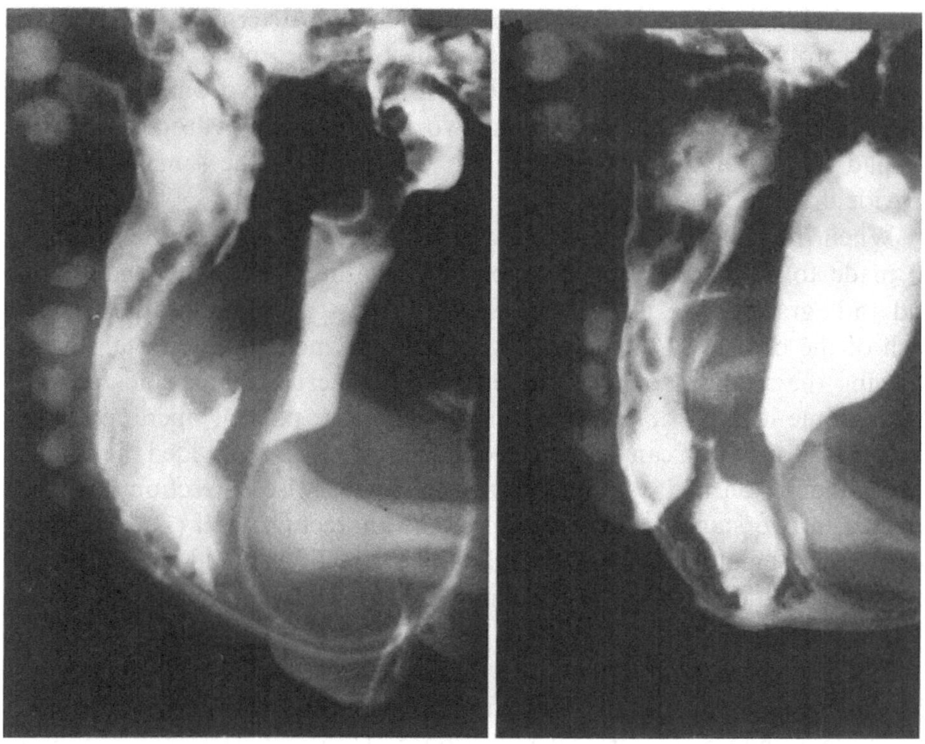

b

Preoperative radiographs will not always provide the information necessary for a definitive surgical correction, i.e., the topography of the cloaca or, preferably, the level of the cloacal malformation and its relation to the bladder sphincter and puborectalis muscle. The preservation of a functioning bladder sphincter, which usually is normal in cloaca patients, and the creation of a competent anorectal sphincter apparatus should be the main concern when formulating an operative treatment plan. In this case the general rule that a malformation should be corrected as early as possible and in a single session is occasionally moderated by the consideration that bladder and rectal function are the first priority, while vaginal reconstruction is a secondary concern. This means that a minimum of three sessions are then required:

1. Colostomy
2. Sacral-abdominal-perineal pullthrough to correct the rectal malformation
3. Vaginoplasty

As stated above, preoperative studies do not always demonstrate the topography of the cloaca and associated structures, particularly the rectum in its relation to the puborectalis muscle. Thus, to determine whether the rectum protrudes through the puborectalis sling or enters the cloaca at a higher level, it is necessary first to establish a colostomy from the sigmoid colon to the left lower abdomen. In two patients with hydrometrocolpos we had to pass a Casper catheter into the uterus in the same sitting to provide drainage.

When the child has been doing well for several weeks, an attempt may be made to define the precise topography of the cloaca with endoscopy and radiography. We use an endoscope to pass a ureteral catheter into each of the orifices in the cloaca, inject contrast medium and obtain films showing the relations of the bladder, urethra, uterus, vagina and rectum. At this time it is possible to formulate a definitive plan of operation. The cloacal malformation can be corrected in a single session provided the child's general condition and anatomy permit this; otherwise correction must be effected in two stages: (1) correction of the anorectum; and (2) correction of the vaginal malformation. While the first correction should be performed at about 6 months of age, we recommend that the vaginoplasty be done at 18–24 months.

Hendren (1980, 1983) generally treats the cloacal syndrome by detaching the vagina and rectum from the urethra in one session and performing a complete abdominal perineal pullthrough. However, Hendren does not report any precise figures for manometric measurements documenting the functional results with the anorectal sphincters.

Correction of the rectal malformation is beyond the scope of this book. The techniques practiced at our center, their indications and their results have been published elsewhere by the author and his colleague Holschneider (see References).

Separation of the vagina from the urethra and urogenital sinus is generally done using the abdominoperineal technique described under "Surgical Correction of Urogenital Sinus with High Vaginal Entry." Hendren (1983) recommends that anomalous ureteral drainage and megaloureter be corrected in the same session. We also feel that this is appropriate, provided the child can tolerate the additional surgical stress. If the vaginoplasty proves tedious, it is better to postpone the vesicoureteral surgery for several months.

The great majority of cloacal malformations are located well above the puborectalis muscle. However, low forms in which the rectum and vagina protrude through the puborectalis sling or lie directly within it are occasionally seen. In these situations it is possible to correct the rectal or vaginal malformation in a single session, using a sacroperineal pullthrough to correct the anal and rectal atresia (Fig. 21). The child is positioned prone with the pelvis elevated, and the "anal fossa" (normal anal site) is electrically stimulated to determine the location of the external sphincter. A cruciate incision is made at that site, and four triangular skin flaps are mobilized. Electrical stimulation is again used to find the center of the external sphincter, the muscle is carefully spread apart at that location, and underlying tissues are dissected to a depth of 1–1.5 cm. The wound cavity is packed with a moist patty. A horizontal incision is made over the coccyx, which is then separated from the sacrum. The puborectalis muscle is exposed, the rectum and vagina are dissected free, and the urethra is identified with the aid of a catheter previously passed into the bladder. The dissection is more difficult if the catheter has entered the rectum or vagina. Following separation of the rectum and vagina and their detachment from the urethra, the urethra is repaired, and the rectum is mobilized for pullthrough. Usually this can be done without difficulty. Adequate mobilization of the vagina is more problematic. Frequently the vagina is not long enough to reach the perineum, and the uterus cannot be mobilized from the sacral approach as it can in the abdominoperineal procedure. Two options are available for joining the vagina to the perineum if a direct vaginal pullthrough is not possible: either by the creation of 2 perineal skin flaps as shown in Fig. 12e, h, i and Fig. 13b, c, or by the insertion of a stent from the perineum, as shown in Fig. 13a, b. In either case, adequate access and vision require that the vaginal malformation be corrected before the rectum is pulled through.

After the rectum and vagina have been isolated and the urethra repaired with 5-0 Vicryl, a dressing forceps is introduced through the previously dissected anal fossa into the sacral field until it is visibly within the puborectalis sling. Now a small dressing forceps is passed into the sacral field through a cruciate incision in the perineal region, where the vaginal opening is normally located. This creates a channel into which a stent is inserted as shown in Fig. 13a, b, engaging the vagina. Then the dressing forceps in the anal canal is used to grasp holding sutures in the mobilized rectum and pull the rectum through to the anal fossa, where it is sutured to the skin flaps.

Fig. 21a–d. Surgical correction of the cloacal malformation, sacroperineal technique

Fig. 21a. Top *Cross-sectional view showing a cloacal malformation located in the region of the puborectalis muscle. The rectum is posterior, the bladder and urethra are anterior, and the vagina is at the center.* Bottom *With the child positioned prone, the external anal sphincter is localized by electrical stimulation of the anal fossa (cf. Fig. 22c). A cruciate incision is made at that site, the anal sphincter is dissected, and an incision is made over the coccyx. The plane of the incision is indicated by the* broken line

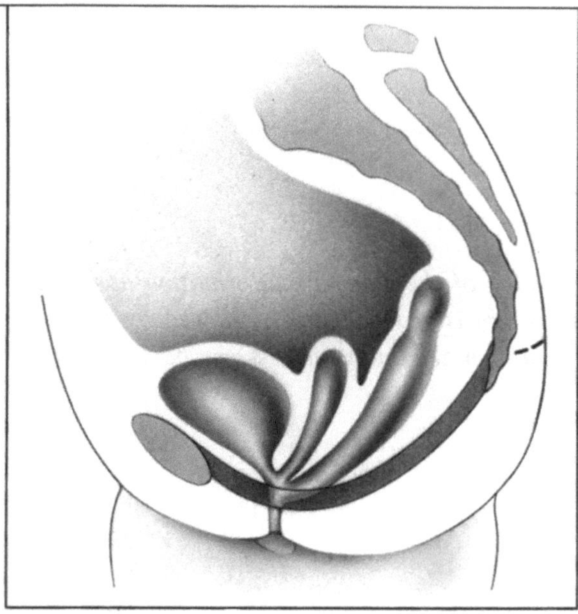

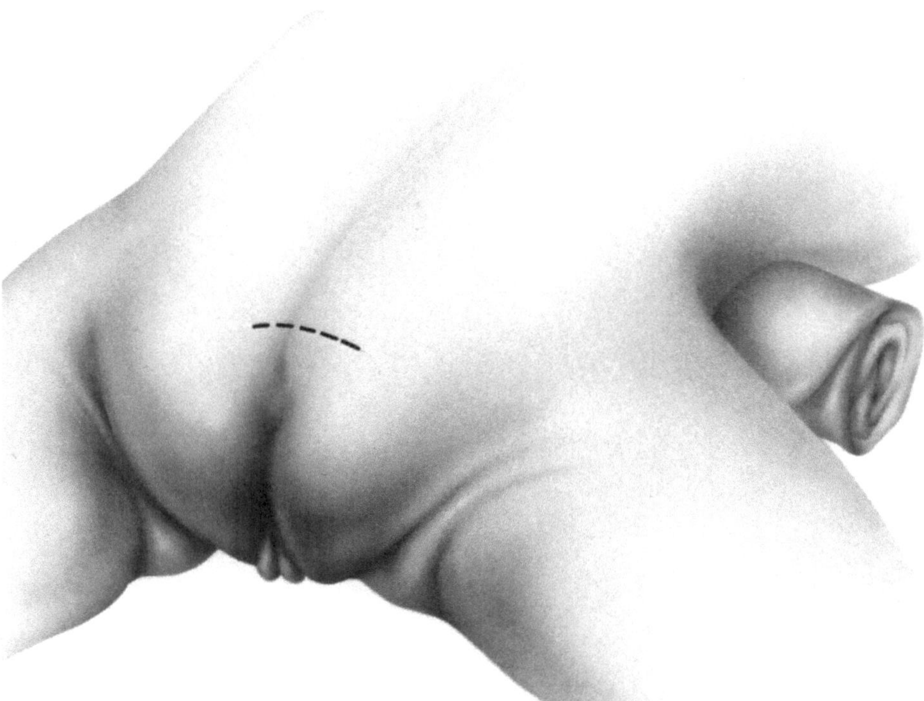

Fig. 21b. Topography of the cloacal malformation as viewed from the sacral approach: The rectum is reached first, followed by the vagina and urethra. The urethra is catheterized and generally can be palpated without difficulty

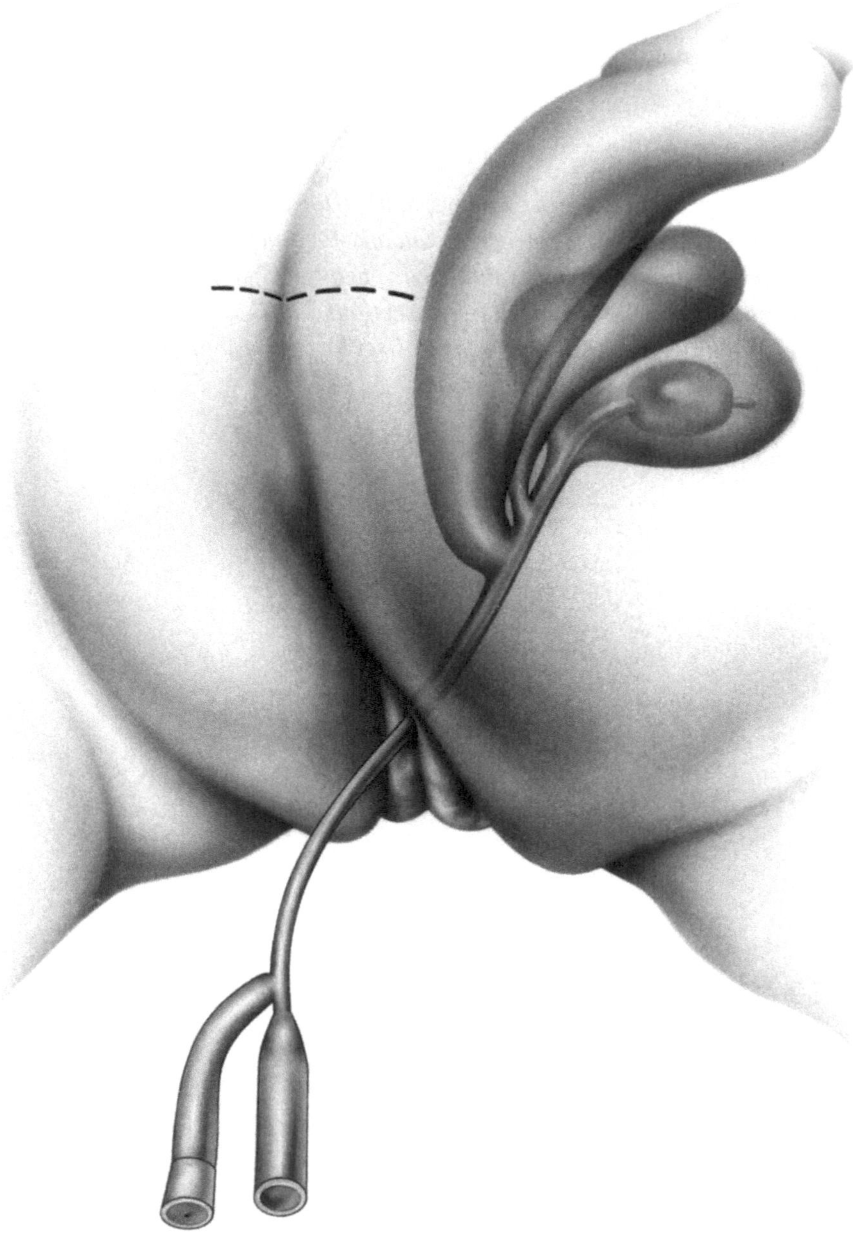

Fig. 21c. Top *Appearance of the coccyx and attached puborectalis fibers.* Bottom *The detached coccyx is retracted caudally together with the puborectalis muscle, which has been carefully mobilized. Then the cloaca, rectum, vagina, and urethra are successively exposed by dissection. This part of the operation is usually very tedious due to the presence of rectovaginal and urethrovaginal adhesions*

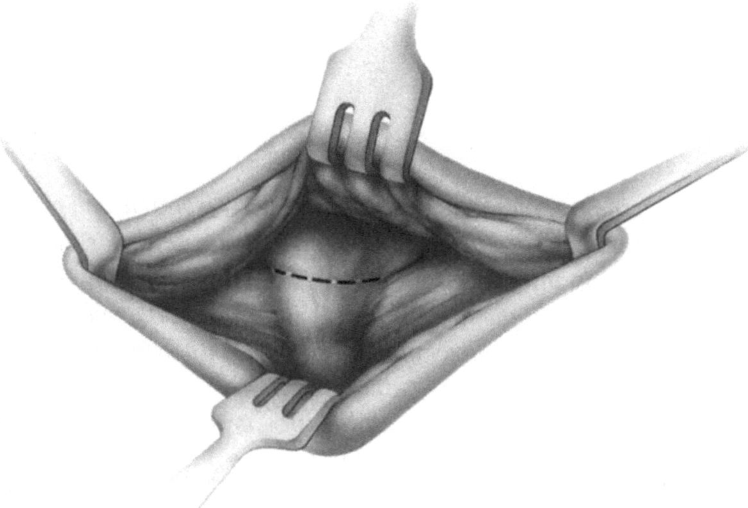

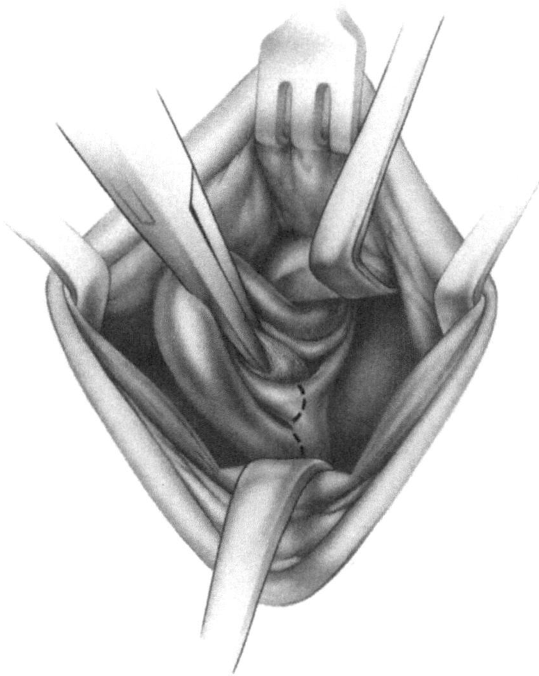

Fig. 21 d. After the vagina, rectum, and urethra have been isolated, the cloacal attachments to the urethra are divided, and the urethral defect is sutured. A small dressing forceps is introduced into the sacral field through the previously dissected anal fossa until the forceps is definitely within the puborectalis sling. Then the previously mobilized rectum is engaged with two stay sutures and pulled through to the anal fossa. Next a cruciate incision is made in the region of the perineum where the vaginal orifice is normally found, and a channel is created through which a vaginal stent is inserted. This stent is fixed as shown in Fig. 13 c and f. The possible ways of constructing a direct connection between vagina and perineum are shown in Figs. 12 and 13

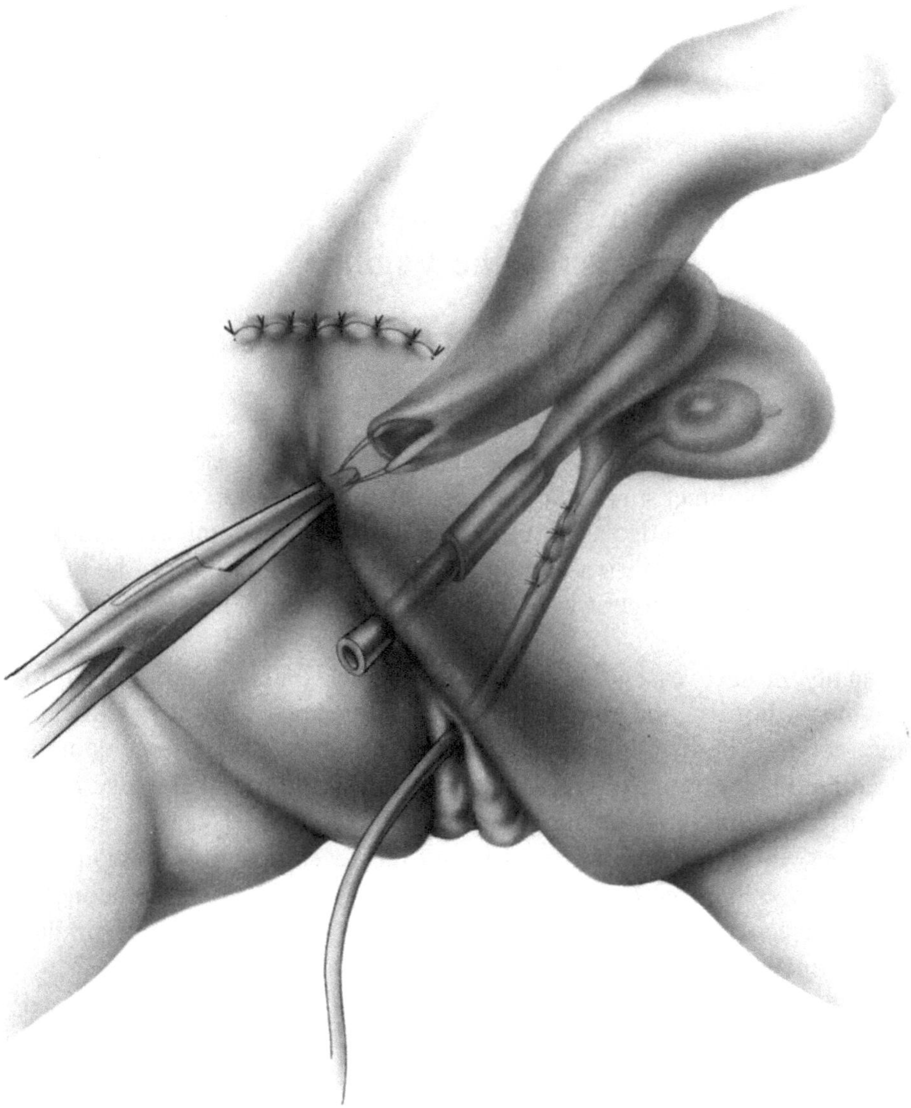

Correction of an Ectopic Anus in the Vestibular Fossa of the Vagina

In high, combined vaginorectal malformations involving rectal atresia with a vaginal fistula, direct surgery of the vagina is not necessary and the fistula is simply underrun and tied as part of a sacral-perineal-abdominal submucosal rectal pullthrough. With a low rectovaginal malformation, on the other hand, direct vaginal surgery is performed according to the technique described below.

Usually in such cases the rectum enters the vagina just posterior to the hymenal border, and the vaginal epithelium merges directly with that of the rectum. The fistulous opening in the rectum is usually large enough to accommodate a No. 5–7 Hegar dilator. During the first 4–6 weeks postpartum the ectopic anal opening is dilated in stages to Hegar 11 so that the patient will be able to defecate without the development of a secondary megarectum. When the child has thrived for 3–4 weeks after the neonatal period, corrective surgery is initiated. We use a technique that is similar to Pott's operation, combining it with a levator plasty (Fig. 22).

The infant is placed in the lithotomy position, and a catheter is passed into the bladder. All operative steps beyond that point should be done with at least a 4 X and preferably a 6 X binocular loupe, which is also worn by assistants. An operating microscope is optional.

The anal fossa and underlying external sphincter are identified by electrical stimulation and incised in cruciate fashion to create four skin flaps that meet at the center. A dissecting scissors is used to make a tunnel at the center of the Sphincter musculature, and this tunnel is enlarged to Hegar 8–10 with a small dressing forceps. A small dissecting patty soaked in saline is placed into the wound.

A semielliptical incision is made 2–3 mm caudal to the ectopic anal opening, following the curve of the labia majora. A microscissors is then used to cut around the anterior border of the ectopic rectal opening, separating it from the vagina. The posterior commissure is dissected free for about 1 mm and engaged with a 6-0 stay suture, which is held with extreme care by an assistant. Further dissection is done with the aid of very fine atraumatic forceps, micropatties, microscissors, fine two- or three-prong hooks, and fine Langenbeck retractors. The rectum is dissected free and mobilized in a staged fashion, making every effort to preserve its relations to the puborectalis sling. When the rectum has been dissected free for a length of 4–5 cm over its anterior wall (vaginal side) as well as posteriorly and laterally in relation to the puborectalis muscle, a very fine dressing forceps or Overholt hemostat is introduced into the perineal field through the previously dissected anal fossa. The rectum is then grasped, pulled through to the fossa, and sutured to the previously mobilized anal skin flaps. The flaps are sutured to the rectum with nonabsorbable 6-0 threads. Next the previously mobilized levator, to which the puborectalis belongs, is joined anterior to the rectum with two or three threads of 5-0 atraumatic Vicryl. This accomplishes two things: It creates a suitable perineal body, and it surrounds the rectum with levator muscle – an important prerequisite for anal competence. In the next step, the posterior portion of the horizontal incision in the posterior vaginal commissure is sutured in a vertical direction with two or three threads to extend the perineum. Then the posterior commissure, which was engaged with stay sutures, is sutured to the perineal skin (6-0 Vicryl). The vagina is packed for 4 days with a small tulle strip, and the wound is sealed with bucrylate. The bladder catheter is removed after 5 days. Both legs are then extended vertically to relieve pressure on the buttocks and keep feces from soiling the perineal wound region. The anal sutures are removed 10 days postoperatively. The sutures for the perineum and posterior commissure consist of 6-0 atraumatic Vicryl.

Fig. 22a. To correct an ectopic anus in the vestibular fossa of the vagina, the anal is first carefully identified by electrical stimulation and marked. A horizontal incision is made caudal to the ectopic anal opening on line with the labia majora and is carried around the ectopic anus at the junction of the vaginal and rectal mucosae. At least a 4X, and preferably a 6X, operating loupe is necessary, for we undertake this procedure in newborns who have thrived for about 6 weeks

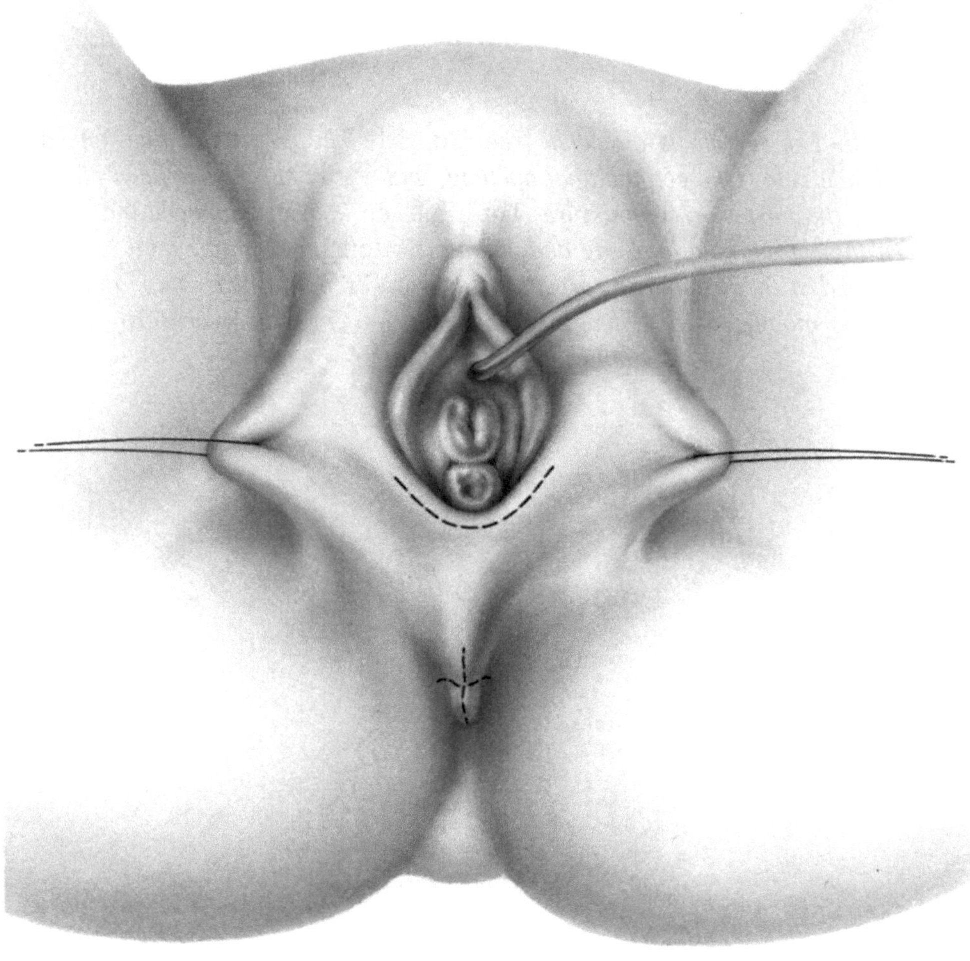

Fig. 22b. The rectum is dissected free. Top left *The horizontal incision has been made below the ectopic anal opening, and a stay suture has been placed through the posterior commissure.* Top right *An incision has been made between the ectopic anal opening and vagina.* Bottom *The ectopic anal opening is grasped with atraumatic forceps (stay sutures might tear out), and the rectum is mobilized for a length of at least 5–6 cm with microscissors and microdissecting patties*

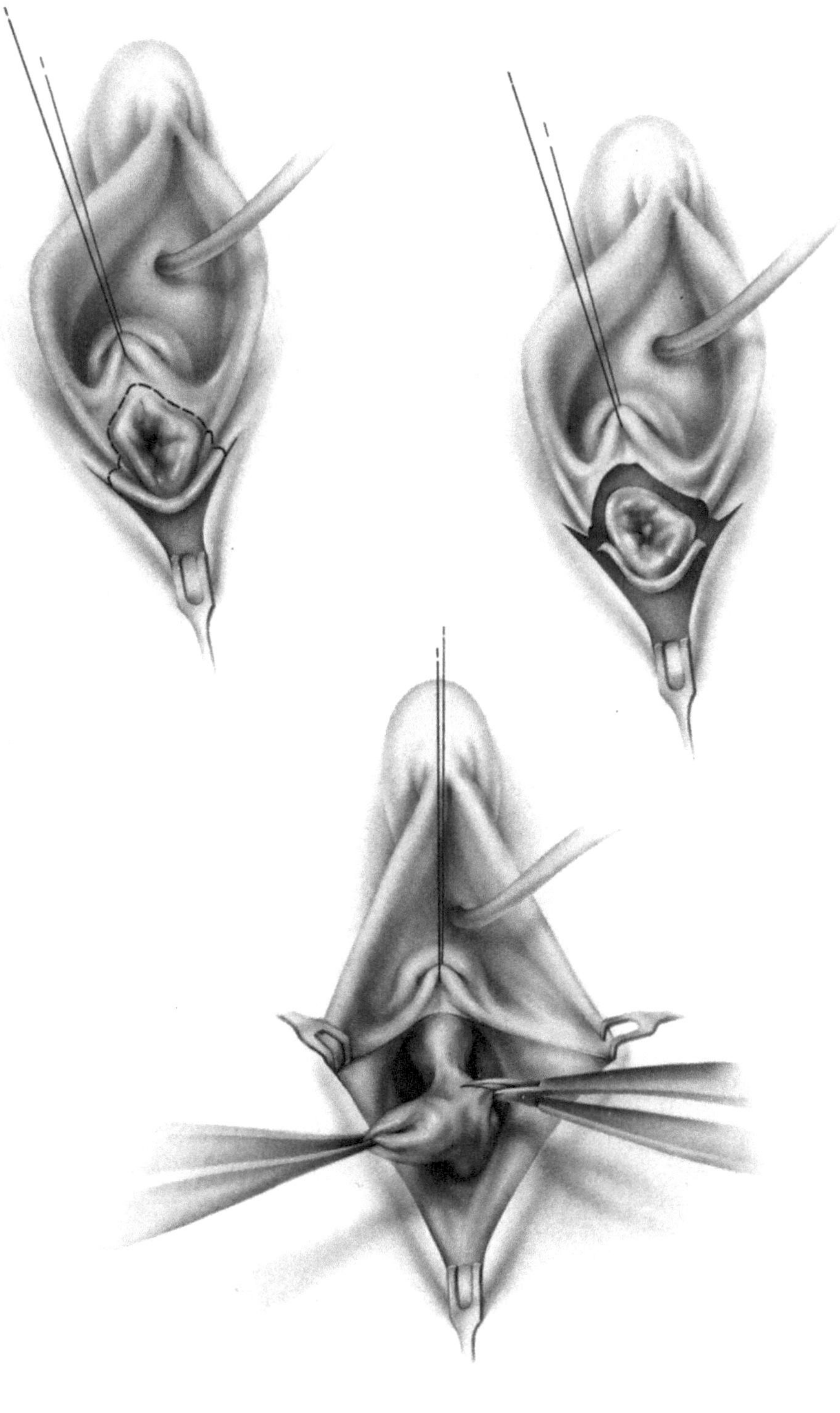

Fig. 22c. Following adequate rectal mobilization, a cruciate incision is made at the anal fossa, and the external anal sphincter is dissected at its center (left). *Then an fine dressing forceps is inserted through the dissected anal fossa and sphincter into the operative field posterior to the vagina, and the mobilized rectum is grasped and pulled through to the anal fossa* (right)

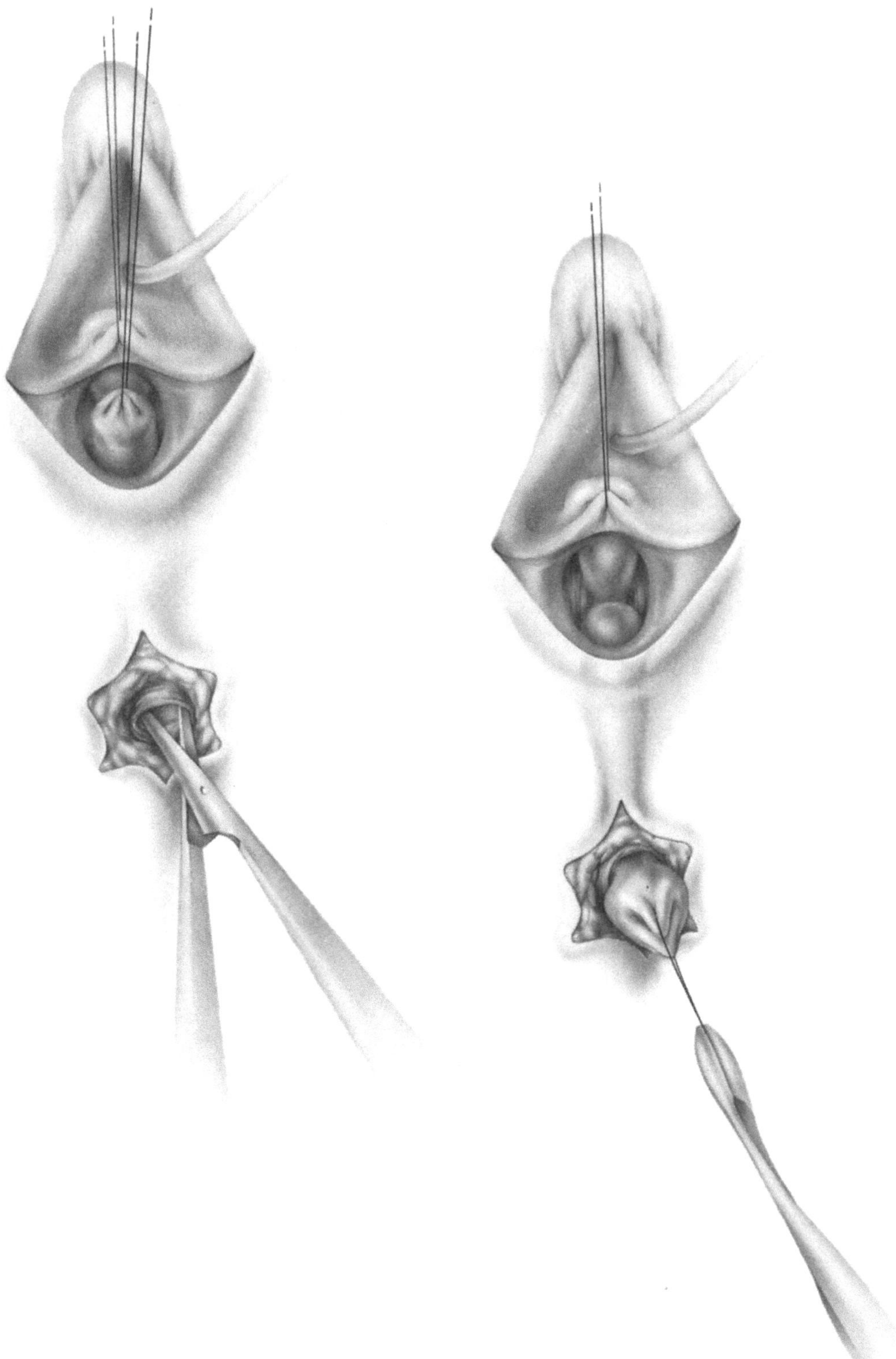

Fig. 22d. Following the pullthrough, the levator branches presenting in the right and left sides of the field are joined over the rectum. The left drawing *shows the placement of the sutures, and the* right drawing *shows the sutures tied. A small suction drain is also shown. The next step is wound closure, which is begun by suturing the primary transverse incision longitudinally to extend the perineum. The lateral parts of the wound are then sutured to the posterior vaginal wall*

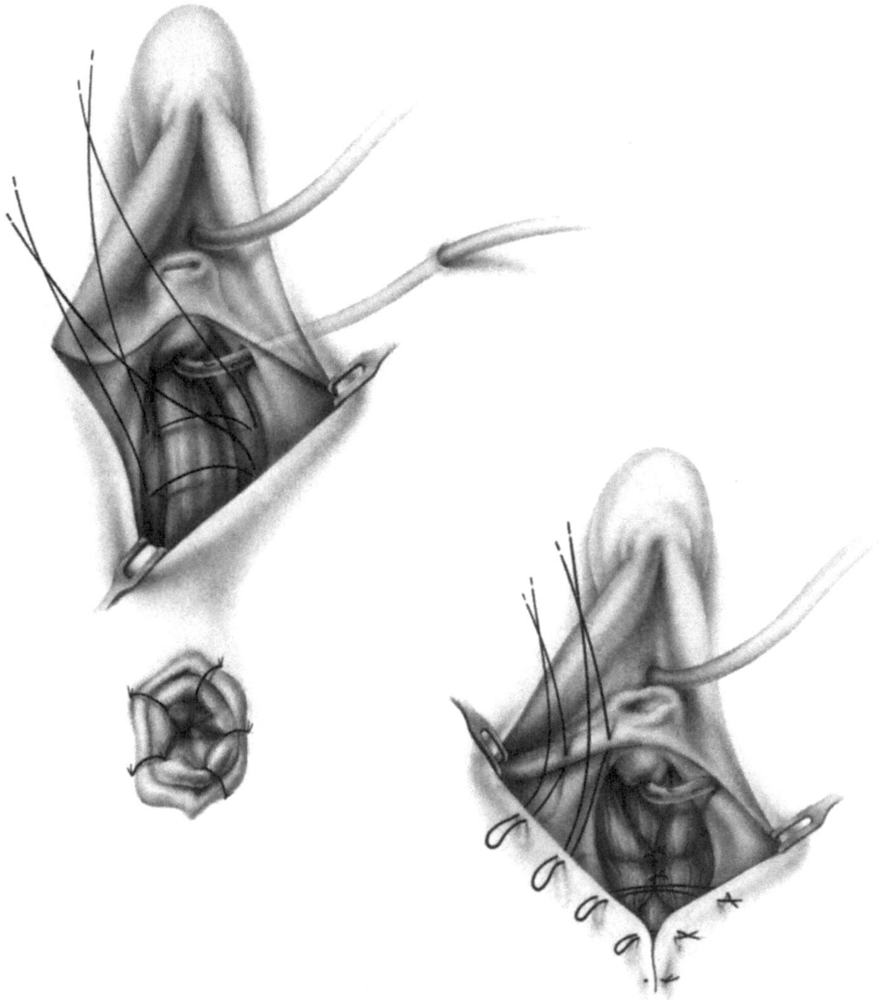

Fig. 22e. The pulled-through rectum is sutured into the anal fossa, and a portion of the primary horizontal incision is sutured vertically to extend the perineum. A bladder catheter is left in place, a small suction drain is inserted into the wound region, and a tulle pack is left within the vagina for 4 days

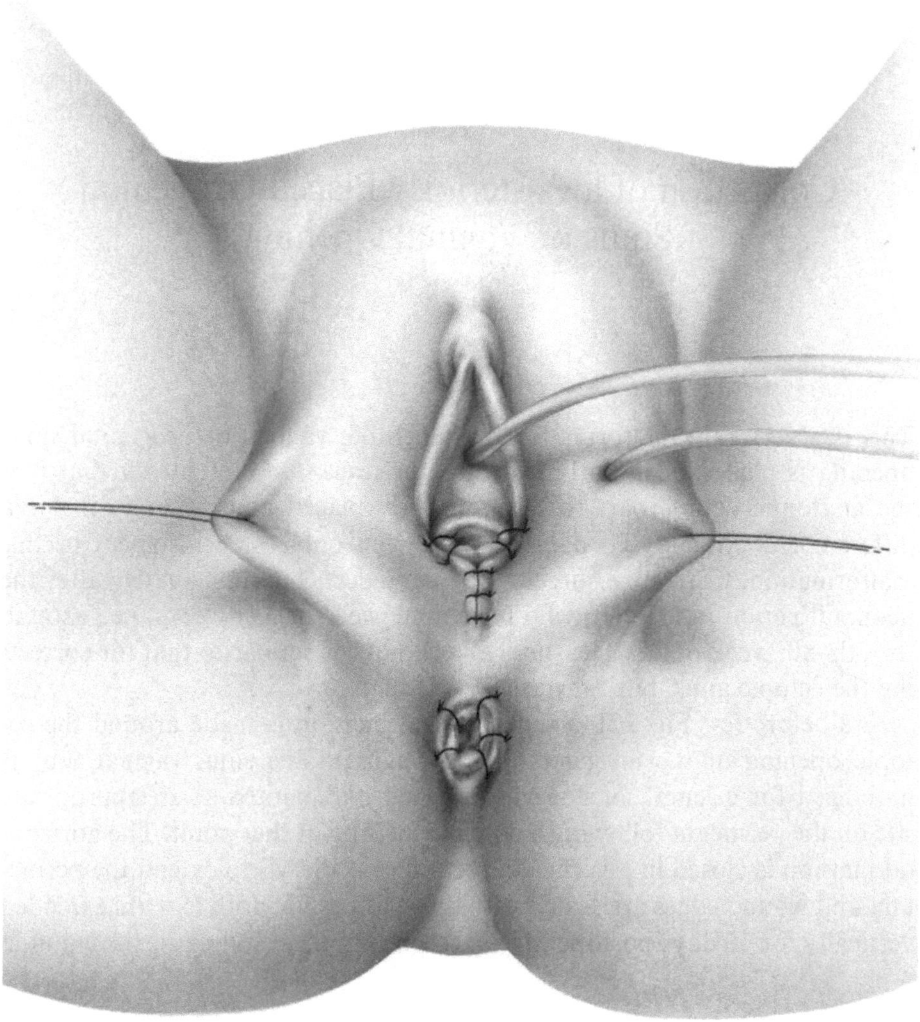

Correction of a Posteriorly Placed Urogenital Sinus or Vaginal Opening

This is a very rare malformation, in which the vaginal or urogenital sinus opening is placed posteriorly, close to the anus. One might say that it is the anatomic counterpart to the anteriorly placed anus, though it has a different embryology. To date we have seen only three instances of this malformation. Corrective surgery may be undertaken immediately after the neonatal period in children who have done well for 3–4 weeks, i.e., around the 6th–8th week of life. The surgical technique is similar to that for correcting the ectopic anus, but "reversed" (Fig. 23).

As before (cf. Fig. 22), a semielliptical incision is made around the ectopic opening of the urogenital sinus (vagina). The sinus/vaginal tube is mobilized for a length of 3–4 cm and then reimplanted at an appropriate site on the perineum following a cruciate incision at that point. The horizontal incision is closed in a vertical direction (6-0 Vicryl) to extend the perineum, and wound edges are sealed with tissue adhesive. Both legs are extended vertically for 10 days postoperatively to prevent fecal soiling of the wound.

→

Fig. 23a. To correct a posteriorly placed urogenital sinus opening, first the bladder is catheterized and filled, and the urine is diverted via a cystotomy (Cystofix)

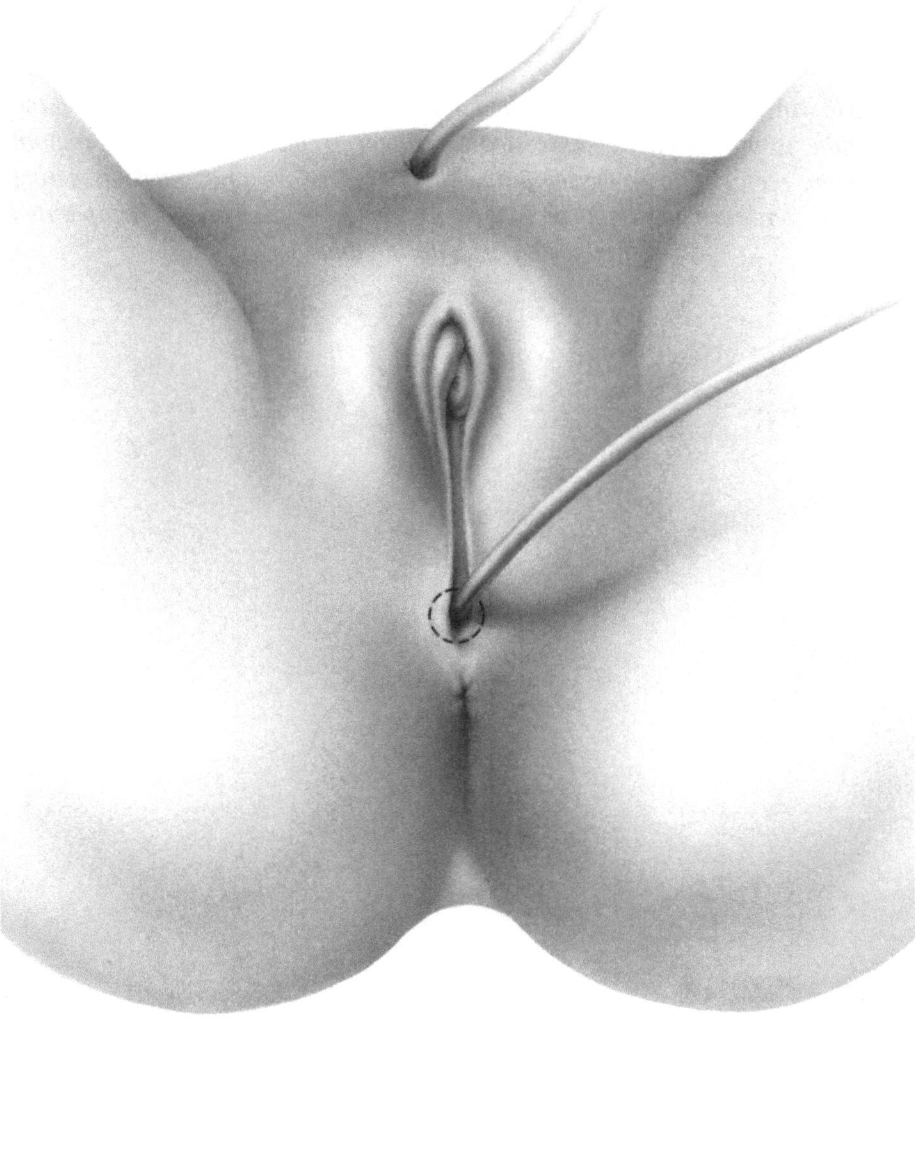

Fig. 23b. An incision is made around the urogenital sinus opening, and the sinus tube is mobilized by dissection. A finger is inserted into the rectum to prevent rectal injury. Dissection with microscissors and microdissecting patties is continued until the mobilized urogenital sinus can be reimplanted farther anterior to the anus

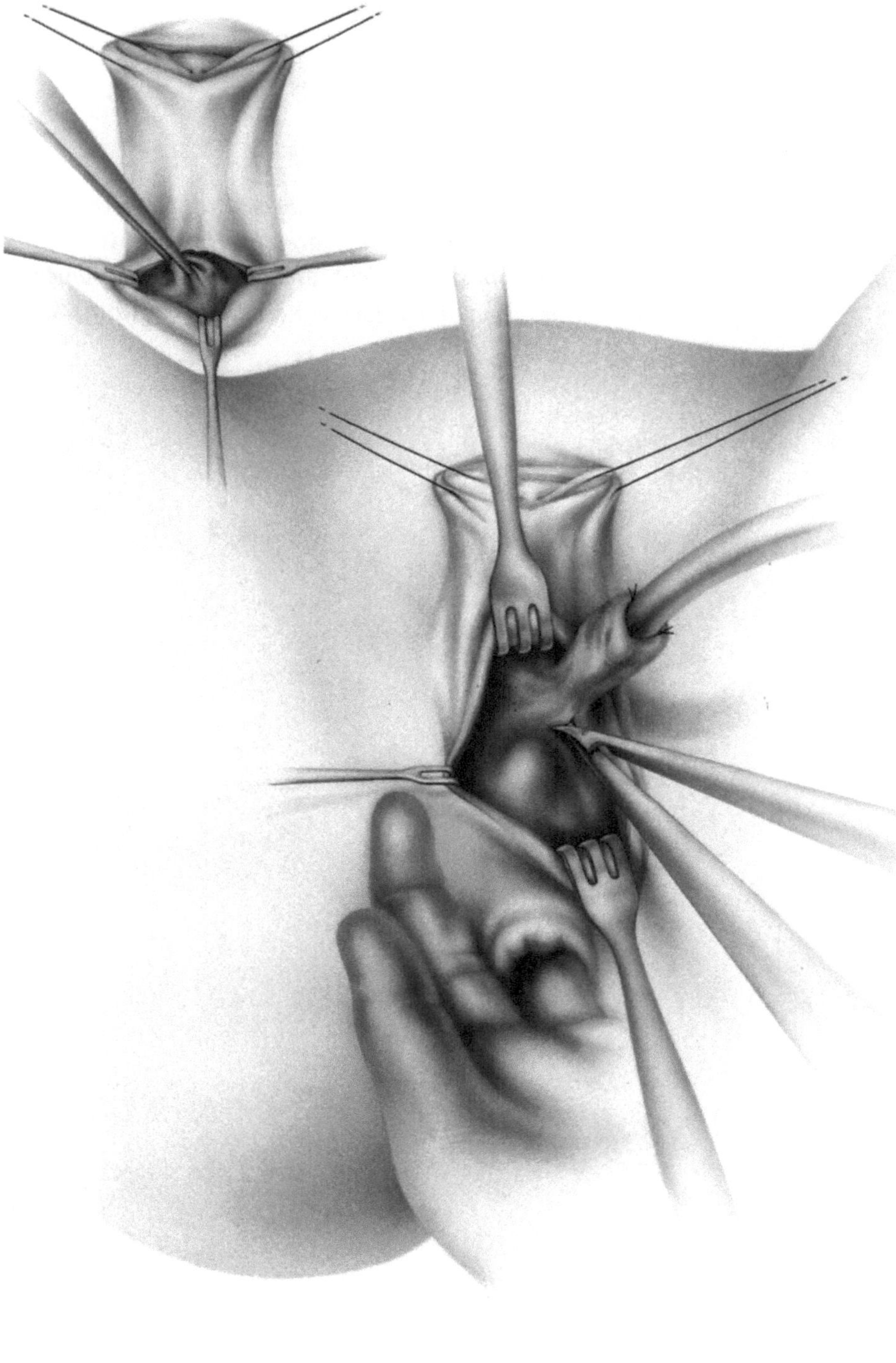

Fig. 23c. Following the mobilization, the skin is incised at the level of the proposed reimplantation (top left), *and a fine dressing forceps is inserted through the incision into the lower operative field. The urogenital sinus opening is grasped by stay sutures and pulled through cranially* (bottom)

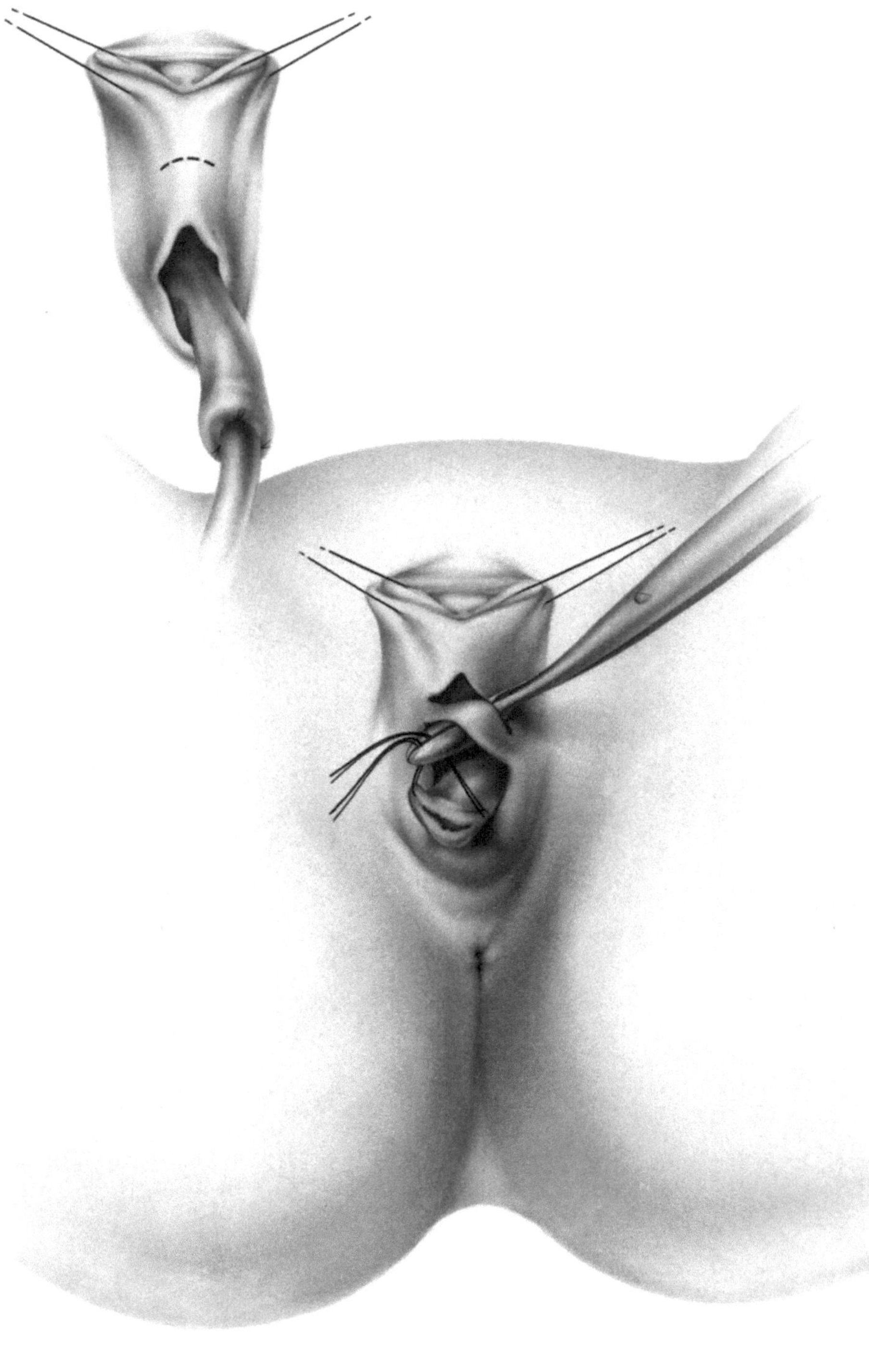

Fig. 23d. The incision around the ectopic urogenital sinus is sutured vertically to elongate the perineum, and the sinus opening is sutured into its new site with 6–0 Vicryl. Urinary diversion by the cystostomy is maintained for 1 week. Both legs are extended in vertical traction, as shown in Fig. 10, to prevent fecal soiling of the wound

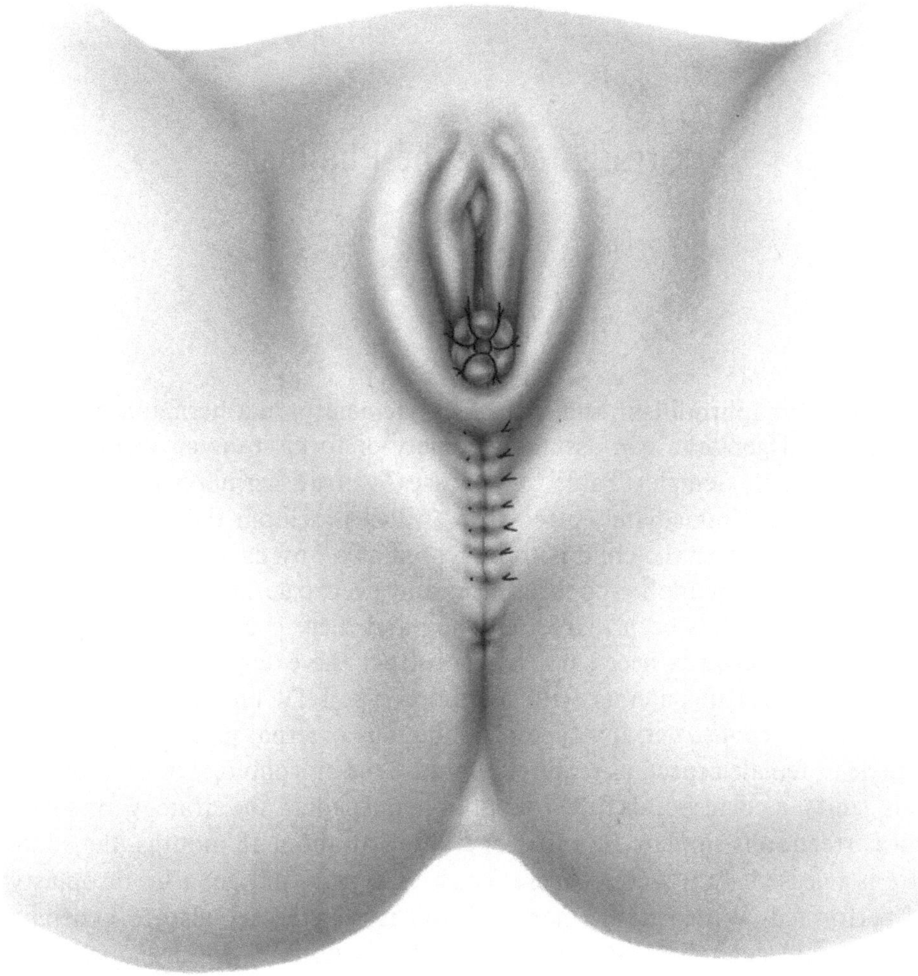

Straightening the Phallus

In true hermaphroditism and in male or female pseudohermaphroditism, the external genitalia can assume a variety of forms ranging from purely male to purely female (Table 1). In cases of true hermaphroditism that are recognized immediately after birth (which is seldom the case), it must be decided whether the child is to be reared as a boy or a girl. In unrecognized cases of pseudohermaphroditism and even true hermaphroditism in which the child has been reared as a boy and there is a desire to maintain that role, it becomes necessary to reconstruct the external genitalia along masculine lines in pateints with a Prader type I–IV anatomy. Today we are able to reconstruct any type of ambigious external genitalia to obtain a male or female aspect, as required. Because the morphology of the ambiguous genitalia corresponds fully to that of hypospadias, the strategy for surgical correction is similar: In a first operation, at about 18 months, the chordee is released. In a second operation, at 3–6 years of age, a urethroplasty is performed. With true hermaphroditism it is necessary also to extirpate the internal genitalia and gonads, and this is done in a third operation. The same applies to female pseudohermaphroditism, in which the vagina, uterus, and ovaries are removed. In a fourth operation, at about 8–9 years of age, testicular prostheses are implanted into the scrotal region of true hermaphrodites and female pseudohermaphrodites.

The straightening operation (Fig. 24) is begun by passing a catheter into the bladder and placing a stay suture through the glans. A narrow bridge of skin 7–8 mm wide is extirpated between the glans and the urethral (UG-sinus) orifice. The incision is continued around both sides of the urethral orifice and extended an additional 1–1.5 cm toward the perineum. The penile skin is mobilized laterally, and the urethra is dissected free and mobilized for length of 2–2.5 cm. At this point the fascial bands which fix the phallus ventrally are excised, and the phallus is straightened. The incision is continued partway into the attachment of the prepuce, and the prepuce and shaft skin are mobilized until the defect formed on the ventral side of the phallus can be adequately covered. The mobilized urethra is then sutured to the lowest point of the perineal incision, and the mobilized shaft skin is closed over the defect; the incision is zigzagged to avoid a straight suture line that would be prone to longitudinal contracture. Secretions are drained by inserting a small strip of Penrose drain or small suction drain into the wound bed. The suture material is 6-0 Vicryl.

The stay suture through the glans is engaged with a rubber sling, which is connected by safety pin to a horizontal plaster strip placed at the thoracic outlet. This is done to fix the straightened phallus in a cranially extended position. A light tulle compression dressing is applied to the phallus for 4 days.

Fig. 24a. A stay suture is placed through the glans, and a ventral incision is made outlining a narrow strip of skin from the meatus to the frenulum. The incision is continued into the prepuce 2 mm from the corona, around the meatus, and further 1–1.5 cm toward the perineum

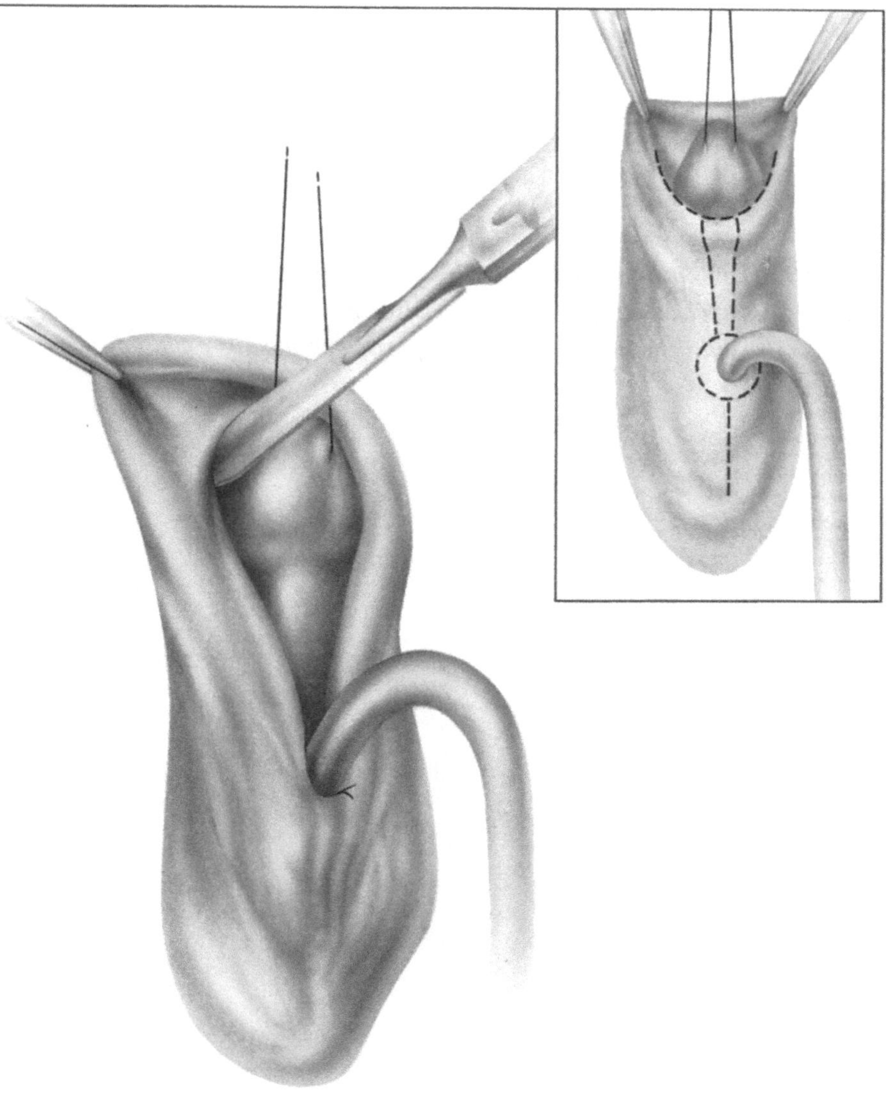

Fig. 24b. The skin is mobilized on all sides, and the fascia binding the penis ventrally is excised. The urethra is dissected free for a length of 1–2 cm, until the division of the corpora cavernosa is exposed

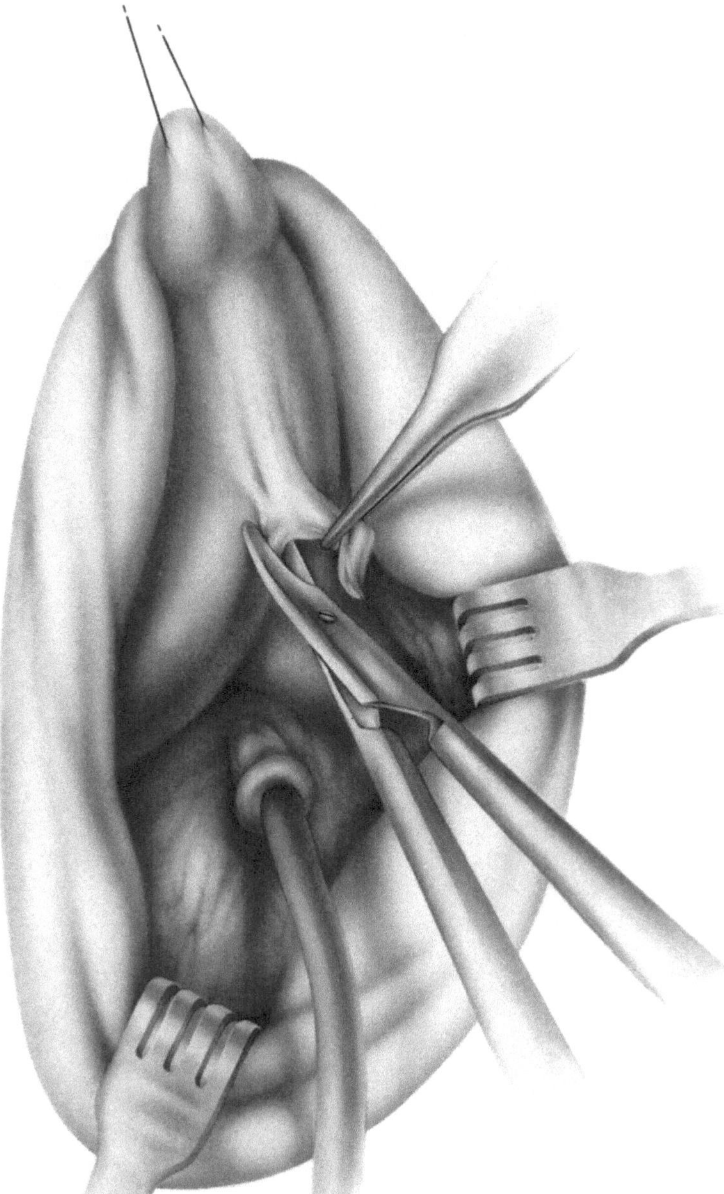

Fig. 24c. Following careful hemostatis and insertion of a drain, a Z is cut at the base of the incision, and the skin is closed with 6–0 Vicryl

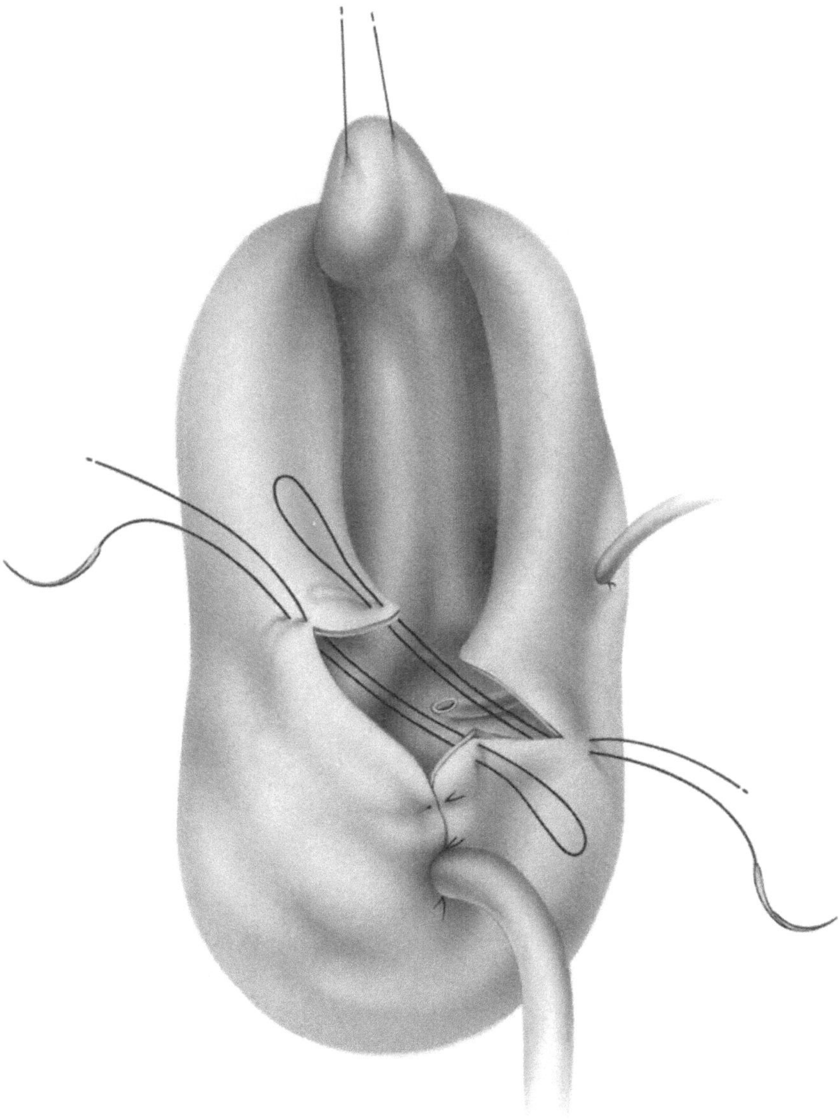

Fig. 24d. The mobilized prepuce is joined to the frenular region of the glans

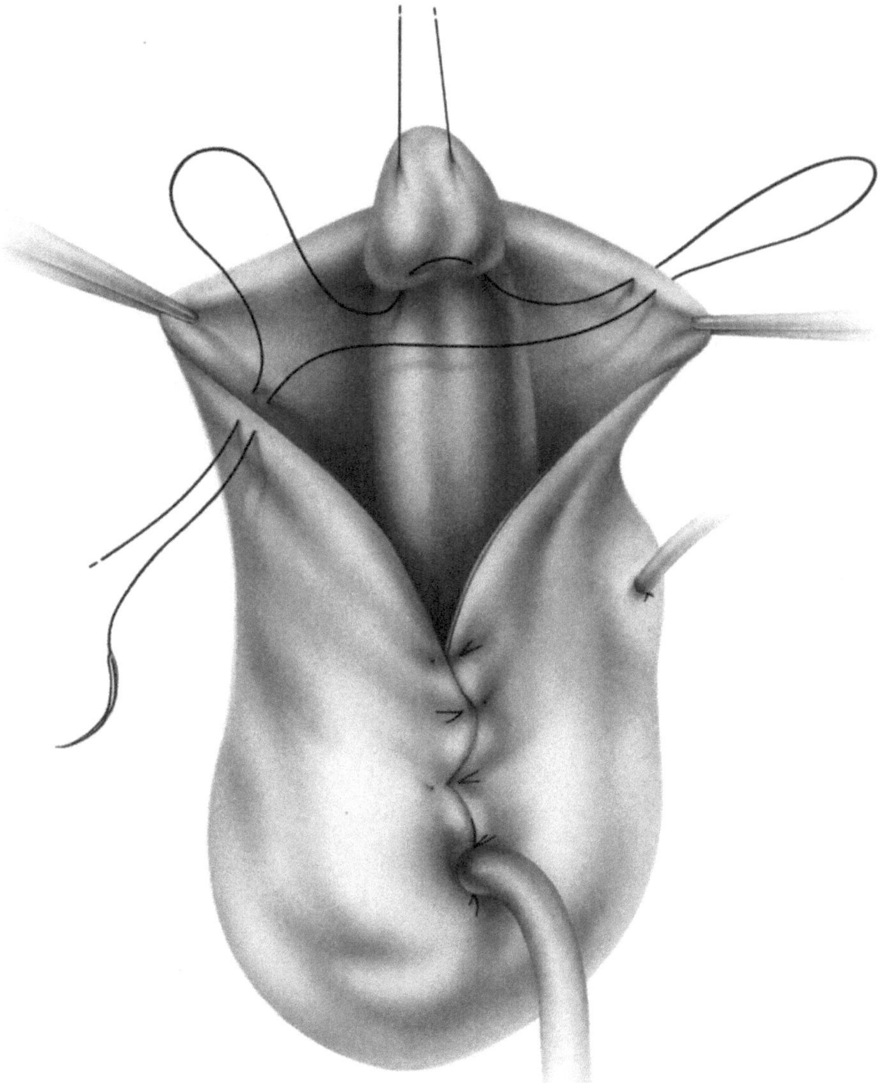

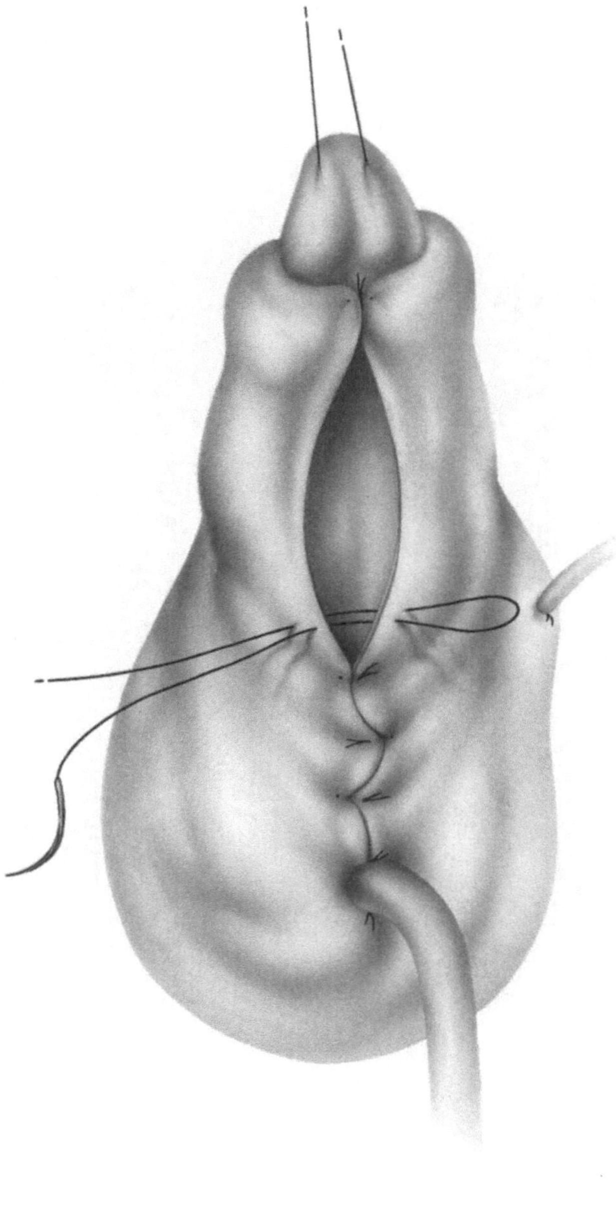

Fig. 24e. Vertical or horizontal mattress sutures are used to obtain good approximation

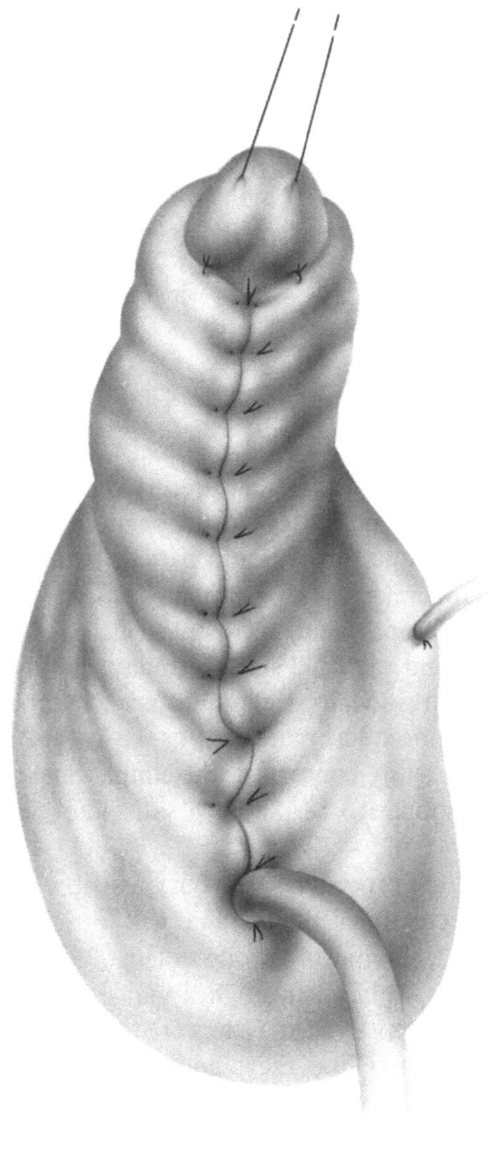

Fig. 24f. Appearance of the penis after the straightening operation

Urethroplasty

All surgical measures to construct a new urethry should be completed before 6 years of age, and thus before the child begins school. In view of the 10–20% incidence of fistula formation in patients who have had a primary urethroplasty, sometimes necessitating as many as four secondary operations to close all the fistulae and recurring fistulae, it is reasonable to perform the urethroplasty around the child's 4th birthday, as this will allow 2 years for secondary procedures. Many techniques are available for construction of a new urethra in hypospadiac patients. For the low forms of hypospadias, with which we are presently concerned, the simple but ingenious technique of Denis Browne continues to be the most satisfactory procedure (Browne 1949).

The basic idea of the procedure is to bury a strip of skin on the ventral aspect of the phyllus, creating a channel that will form a neourethra through epithelialization. Our technique is as follows (Fig. 25):

First a stay suture is placed through a glans. We prefer to use a fine wire suture for this purpose, as it is less irritating than other materials. A Ch 8 catheter is inserted into the bladder, the bladder is filled, and a cystostomy is created to divert the urine (we use the Braun disposable cystostomy set). The operative field should remain completely dry of urine for about 10 days. An incision is then made outlining the "Denis Browne strip," taking care to extend the distal ends of the incision into the tip of the glans and into the prepuce. The lateral skin edges are mobilized together with about one-third of the prepuce on each side, and they are jouned at the midline using a technique suggested by Rehbein (1984); i.e., the wound edges are broadly apposed by means of two narrow-gauge (Ch 5) plastic bolster tubes held in place with mattres sutures (6-0 Ethibond). A strip of Penrose drain is inserted into the wound for temporary drainage and is brought out through a separate stab incision at the penoscrotal junction. Use of the prepuce ensures that the new urethra will extend to the tip of the glans. After the sutures have been placed, a light tulle compression dressing is applied, and the penis is fixed cranially as described in the section on "Straightening the Phallus". The drain is removed on the 1st postoperative day, and the dressing is changed on the 4th–6th day. The sutures and bolster tubes are removed on the 9th postoperative day. The needle tracks will close within 24 h, permitting the cystostomy tube to be removed on the 10th day, at which time the patient may pass urine through his new urethra. Any postoperative fistulae, which usually result from mild wound infection or patent needle tracks, should be closed not less than 6 months after the urethroplasty.

Fig. 25a. Construction of a urethral tube between the meatus and tip of the glans, a median strip of skin on the ventral aspect of the penis is outlined according to the Denis Browne technique. The incision is extended into the tip of the glans and around half the circumference of the prepuce on each side

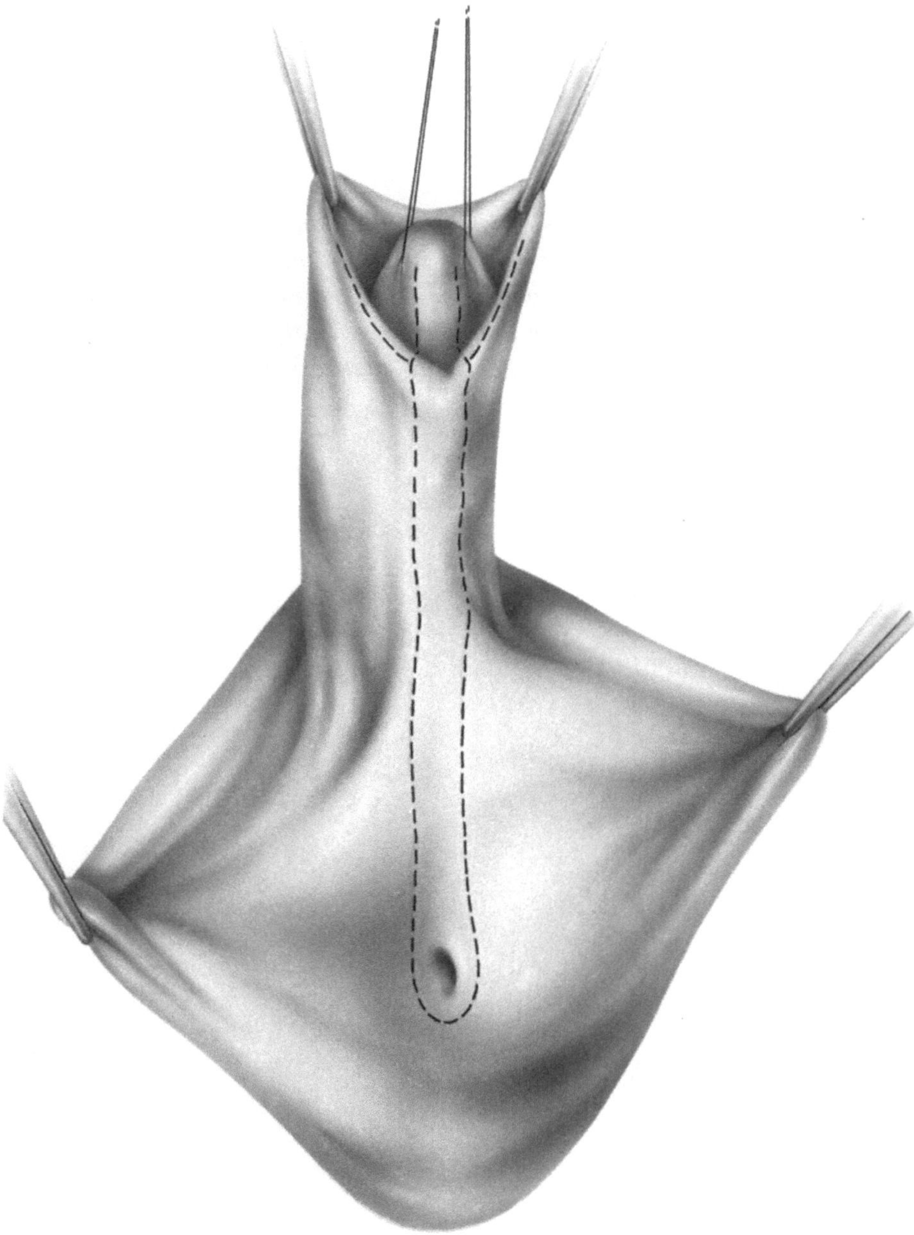

Fig. 25 b. The skin is widely mobilized on all sides and closed over the median strip. The mobilized prepuce is sutured so as to cover the strip out to the tip of the glans. Top right *To obtain broad apposition of the wound edges, two lengths of Ch 5 plastic tubing are laid alongside the skin edges (technique of Rehbein) and tied in place with horizontal mattress sutures (6–0 Ethibond)*

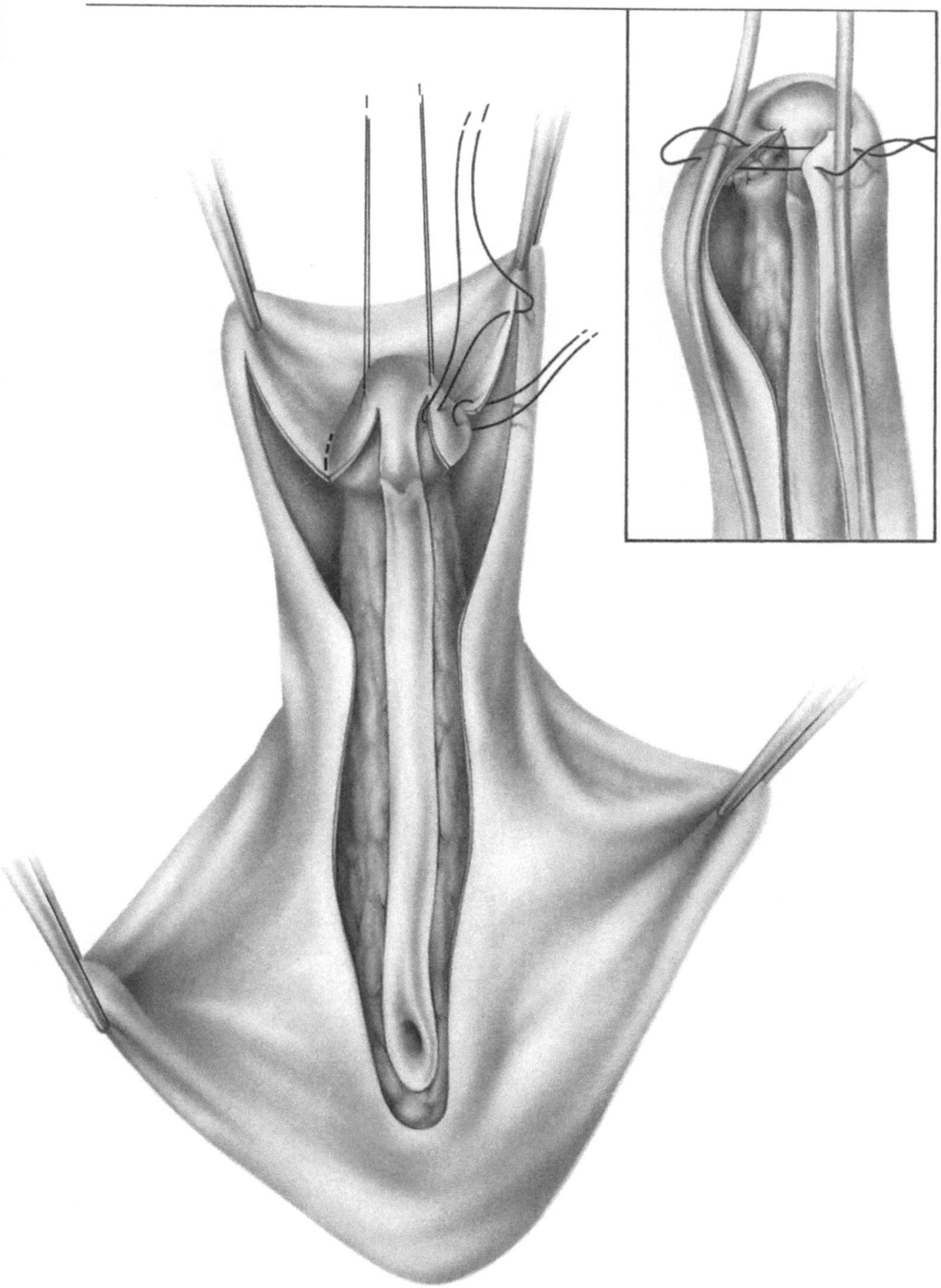

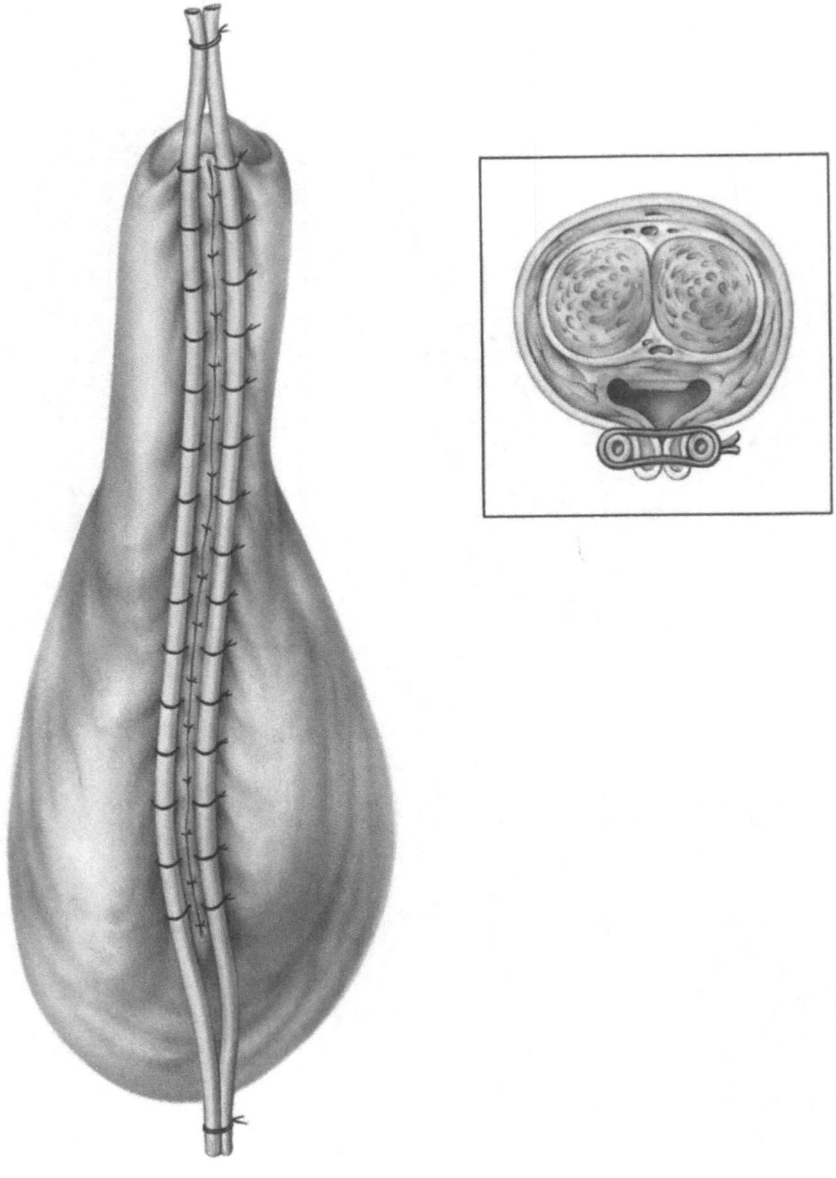

Fig. 25c. The completed urethroplasty using the Denis Browne technique and the Rehbein method of skin closure. Top right *In cross section we see the buried strip over which the skin edges were joined and the broad apposition of the skin edges by the plastic tubes*

Implantation of Prosthetic Testes

There are strong psychological indications for implanting prosthetic testes in children with ambiguous genitals (true hermaphroditism, female pseudohermaphroditism) who are to be reared as males. Of course, these prostheses can be implanted at a very early age, but we prefer to wait until 8 or 9 years of age, since this is the age at which the testes normally begin grow and become conspicuous. A prosthesis of definitive size can the be selected. If it should later prove necessary or desirable to replace the prosthesis with a larger one this can be done without undue difficulty. Usually a sufficient amount of scrotal skin will be available to accomodate the prostheses. However, we strongly recommend that the testes be implanted in two separate operations, allowing an interval of about 3 months before the second prosthesis is inserted. If both prostheses are implanted simultaneously into the hypoplastic scrotum the resulting skin tension may be sufficient to cause necrosis. Our technique is as follows (Fig. 26):

The scrotum is approached through a low, horizontal inguinal incision. Using scissors and patty dissection, a cavity large enough to accept the prosthesis without significant tension is formed in the scrotum. Then, using the index finger, the scrotum is evaginated through the skin incision, and the prosthesis is attached to the exposed tunica dartos with a 4–0 Vicryl suture. The finger is then slowly withdrawn, allowing the prosthesis to slide down into the prepared "scrotal cavity". The inlet of the scrotum is closed with a 3–0 Vicryl pursestring suture to prevent cranial migration of the prosthesis. The wound is closed with subcutaneous sutures and an intracutaneous skin suture. This is a fairly minor procedure which generally can be done under office conditions. We have experienced no wound healing problems, except in earlier cases where an attempt was made to implant both prostheses in a single session.

Fig. 26a. A 3- to 4-cm-long incision is made above the tuberculum pubicum (top right). *Then scissors, patties, and the finger are used to create a bed for the prosthetic testis. The middle finger of one hand is inserted deep into the wound, and the middle finger of the other hand is placed against the outpouched skin and evaginates it out through the incision*

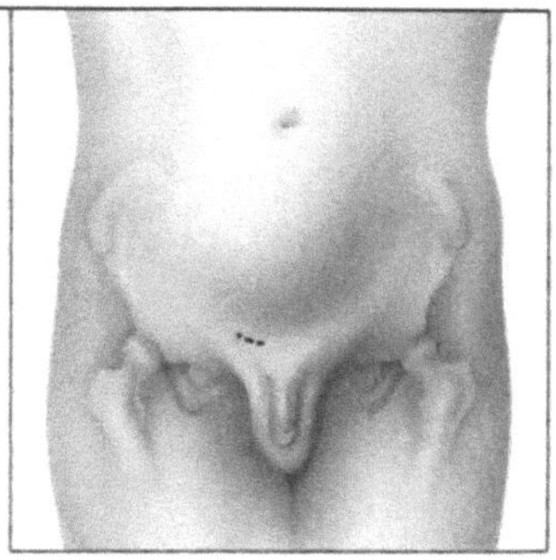

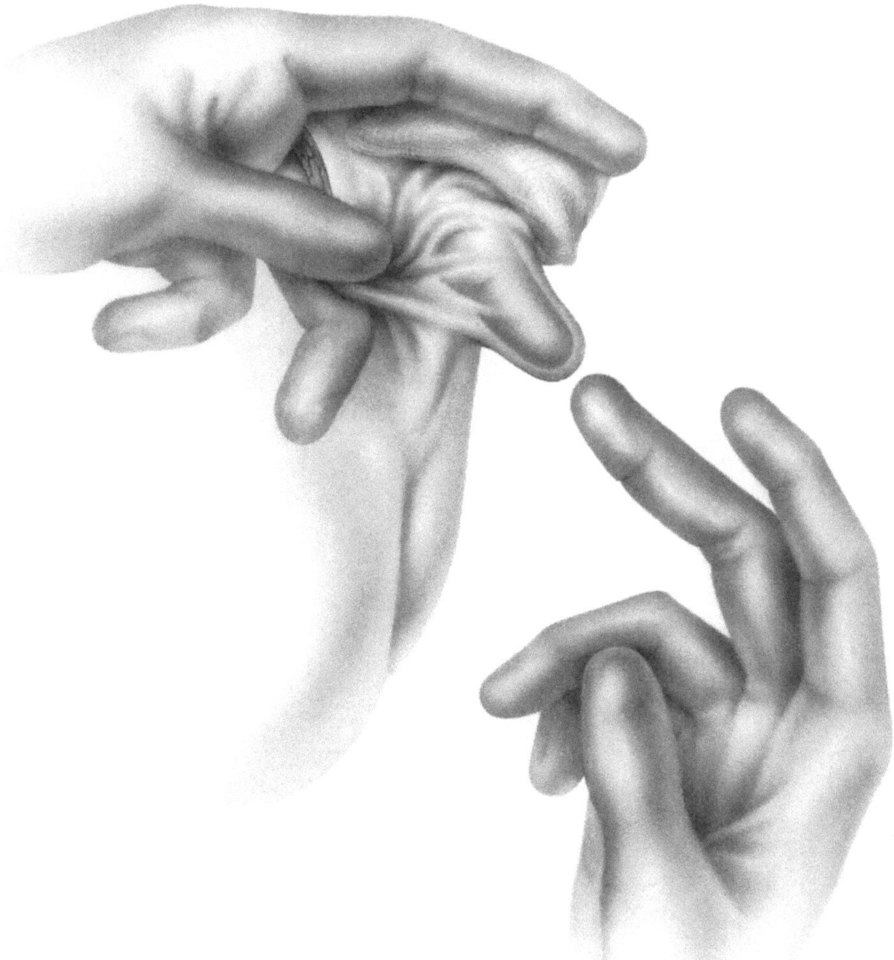

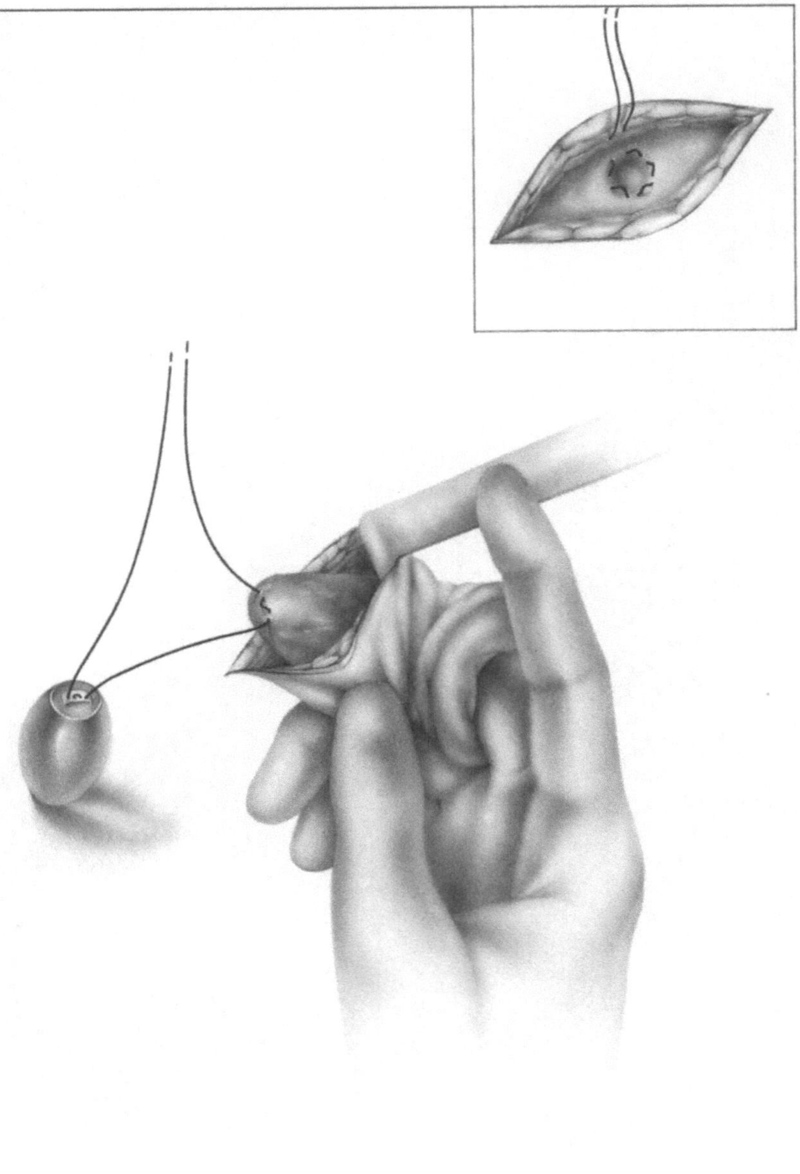

Fig. 26b. The prosthetic testis is sutured to the tunica dartos (bottom), *and the evaginating finger is withdrawn, allowing the prosthesis to slip down into the lowest part of the scrotal sac. The "scrotal inlet" is sealed with a purse-string suture* (top) *to prevent prosthetic migration*

Meatotomy of Prader Type IV Intersexual Genitals Following a Pullthrough Vaginoplasty

A meatotomy is required in a great many patients with Prader type IV genitalia and a high sinovaginal confluence, because the position of the meatus directly below the glans clitoris, which "looks" craniad following plication and recession, also causes the urinary stream to be directed cranially during voiding. These patients have great difficulty urinating in the normal sitting position without staining their clothes. A meatotomy is indicated in these cases to redirect the urinary stream forward and downward. For the operation (Fig. 27) we introduce a grooved probe into the urethra and incise the meatus over the probe the desired distance toward the perineum. The urethral epithelium is then joined to the cutaneous epithelium with 6–0 or 7–0 Vicryl sutures. A bladder catheter is inserted and left in place for 24 h.

Fig. 27a. To perform a meatotomy following clitoroplasty in a Prader type IV individual, a grooved protector is inserted into the urethra, and the ventral part of the urethra is incised with a scalpel so that the urinary stream will be directed forward and downward, rather than cranially, while in the sitting position

Fig. 27b, c. The skin is joined to the urethral epithelium with mattress sutures, and the bladder is catheterized

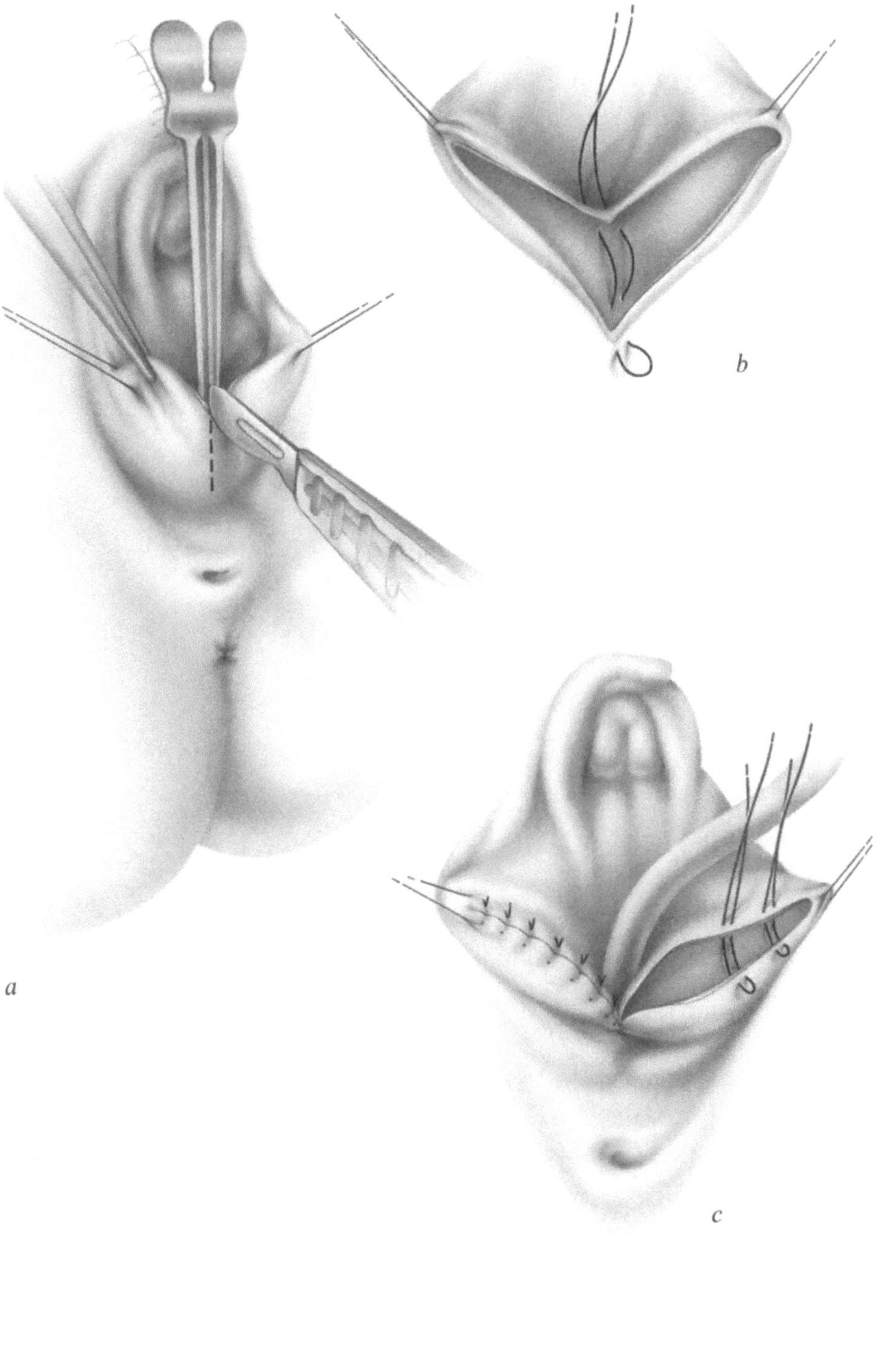

a b c

General Concluding Remarks

Corrective surgery is only one part of the overall management of patients with intersexual or malformed female genitalia. It is equally important that the patient and his parents be properly counseled, that regular follow-up examinations be scheduled to ensure that all anatomical features are growing at the proper rate, and that prompt secondary corrections be undertaken as required. Because a large percentage of these patients have endocrine disorders in addition to their anatomical malformations, life-long endocrinologic supervision and therapy is an integral part of the overall treatment plan.

Experience has shown that these cases are best managed through the cooperative efforts of four specialists – the pediatric surgeon, the pediatric endocrinologist, the child psychologist, and of course, the family pediatrician. At the Dr. von Hauner Pediatric Hospital, we have also found it convenient to keep a single medical record for each patient so that notations made by one physician will be readily available for the rest to see. Whenever surgery is contemplated a meeting is held among the surgeon, endocrinologist, and pediatrician, possibly in the presence of the child psychologist. In addition, regular consultations are held with the parents and patients in which points of importance are explained and clarified, and the parents and older patients have the opportunity to ask questions and verbalize problems of a general nature. Dialogue between parents and discussions among the parents of different patients are also encouraged.

References

Ansell JS, Rajfer J (1981) Hypertrophied clitoris. J Pediatr Surg 16:681

Bolkenius M, Daum R (1977) Verbesserte Methode zur operativ-plastischen Korrektur der Klitoris beim Pseudohermaphroditus femininus. Z Kinderchir 20:71

Browne D (1949) Operation von Hypospadias. Proc R Soc Med 42:466

Cali RW, Pratt JH (1968) Congenital absence of the vagina. Am J Obstet Gynecol 100:752

Counseller VS (1948) Congenital absence of the vagina. JAMA 136:861

Engert J (1983) Eine „Physiologische" Korrektur der virilisierten weiblichen Genitale beim AGS. Chir Prax 31:517

Flach A (1977) Die plastische Korrektur des äußeren weiblichen Genitale im Kindesalter. Z Kinderchir 21:169

Hecker WC (1972) Operative Korrektur bei Differenzierungsstörungen des Sinus Urogenitalis mit Klitorishypertrophie. Chirurg 43:90

Hecker WC (1978) Chirurgische Eingriffe am kindlichen weiblichen Genitale. Fortschr Med 96:604

Hecker WC (1982a) Möglichkeiten der operativen Korrektur des intersexuellen Genitale. In: Hellbrügge T (ed) Die Entwicklung der kindlichen Sexualität. Urban & Schwarzenberg, München Wien Baltimore

Hecker WC (1982b) Zum Zeitpunkt und zur Technik der operativen Korrektur des kindlichen intersexuellen Genitale einschließlich dem Vorgehen bei partieller Vaginalaplasie. Z Kinderchir 37:93

Hecker WC (1982c) Rekonstruktion und Konstruktion eines schlußfähigen Anus naturalis bei fehlgebildeten Kindern. Chirurg 53:616

Hecker WC (1984) Operative correction of intersexual genitalis in children. Prog Pediatr Surg 17:21

Hecker WC, Holschneider AM (1983) Sacro-perineo-abdominelles Vorgehen bei hoher Anal- und Rektumatresie. In: Hofmann-v. Kapp-her, S. (ed) Ano-rektale Fehlbildungen. Fischer, Stuttgart New York

Hemminger H (1982) Verhaltensbiologische Grundlagen der kindlichen Sexualentwicklung. In: Hellbrügge T (ed) Die Entwicklung der kindlichen Sexualität. Urban & Schwarzenberg, München Wien Baltimore

Hendren WH (1980) Urogenital sinus and anorectal malformation. J Pediatr Surg 15:628

Hendren WH (1983) Further experience in reconstructive surgery for cloacal anomalies. J Pediatr Surg 17:695
Hendren WH, Crawford JD (1969) Adrenogenital syndrome. J Pediatr Surg 4:49
Hendren WH, Donalire PK (1980) Correction of congenital abnormalities of the vagina and perineum. J Pediatr Surg 15:751
Hienz HA (1969) Intersexuelle Störungen der Geschlechtsentwicklung. Fortschr Med 87:484
Kirschner M, Wagner GA (1930) Ein neues Verfahren der künstlichen Scheidenbildung. Zentralbl Gynäkol 54:2690
Marberger M, Marberger H, Stockamp K, Straub E (1975) Die Korrektur des intersexuellen Genitale in die weibliche Richtung. Aktuel Urol 6:99
McIndoe AH, Banister JB (1938) An operation for the cure of congenital absence of the vagina. J Obstet Gynaecol Br Commonw 45:490
Prader A (1954) Der Genitalbefund bei Pseudohermaphroditus femininus. Helv Paediatr Acta 9:231
Rehbein F (1984) Androgynie. (Paper presented at the Symposium on Pediatric Surgery, 25.02.1984, Hamburg)
Stefan H (1966) Chirurgische Behandlung des äußeren weiblichen Genitale beim weiblichen Pseudohermaphroditus. Z Kinderchir 3:249
Wharton LR (1938) A simple method of constructing a vagina. Ann Surg 107:842